ALSO BY DR. VICTORIA ZDROK

The Anatomy of Pleasure

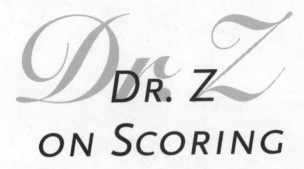

DR. Z
ON SCORING

*How to Pick Up, Seduce, and
Hook Up with Hot Women*

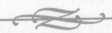

DR. VICTORIA ZDROK

Fireside
A Division of Simon & Schuster, Inc.
1230 Avenue of the Americas
New York, NY 10020

First Fireside trade paperback edition January 2008

FIRESIDE and colophon are registered trademarks of Simon & Schuster, Inc.

For information about special discounts for bulk purchases, please contact Simon & Schuster Special Sales at 1-800-456-6798 or business@simonandschuster.com.

Designed by Jessica Shatan Heslin/Studio Shatan, Inc.

Manufactured in the United States of America

10 9 8 7 6 5 4 3 2 1

Library of Congress Cataloging-in-Publication Data
Zdrok, Victoria Alexandrovna, 1973–.
  Dr. Z on scoring : how to pick up, seduce, and hook up with hot women / by Victoria Zdrok.
    p. cm.
  1. Man-woman relationships. 2. Sex—Handbooks, manuals, etc. 3. Men—Sexual behavior. 4. Interpersonal attraction. 5. Intimacy (Psychology). I. Title.
HQ801.Z38 2008
646.7'7081—dc22
2007024899

ISBN-13: 978-1-4165-5155-3
ISBN-10:   1-4165-5155-7

CREDITS

The photographs of the following Penthouse Pets are used by special permission of General Media Communications, Inc., a subsidiary of Penthouse Media Group Inc.:

- Heather Vandeven: 2007 Pet of the Year; photo by Richard Avery, first published in December 2005
- Jamie Lynn: 2006 Pet of the Year; photo by Ken Marcus, first published in December 2004
- Natalia Cruze: 2005 Pet of the Year Runner-up; photo by Holly Randall, first published in October 2002
- Aria Giovanni: July 2006 cover photo by Mark Mann; first published in August 2000
- Courtney Taylor: 2004 Pet of the Year Runner-up; photo by Carl Wachter, first published in January 2002
- Julie Strain: 1993 Pet of the Year; June 1991 cover photo by Suze Randall, first published in August 1991
- Brea Lynn: November 2006 Pet of the Month; photo by Earl Millen, first published in October 2006
- Erica Ellyson: January 2007 Pet of the Month; photo by Mark Lit for Hicks Photos, first published in December 2006
- Taylor Wane: June 1994 Pet of the Month; photo by Laurien, first published in December 2006
- Krista Ayne: 2007 Pet of the Year Runner-up; photo by Rachael Durz, first published in April 2007

Tatiana Zdrok, Penthouse model: Photo by Cynthia Kaye

Charlotte Kemp, Miss December 1982: Photo by John Perrige, owned by Charlotte J. Helmkamp

Art by Dan Thompson

Contents

Introduction

The first thing to get in your head is that every single
Girl can be caught—and that you'll catch her if
You set your toils right. Birds will sooner fall dumb in
Springtime, cicadas in summer, or a hunting-dog
Turn his back on a hare, than a lover's bland inducements
Can fail with a woman. Even one you suppose reluctant
Will want it.   —OVID, *The Art of Love*

Men play the game; women know the score. —ROGER WODDIS

SCORING

You walk into a party, a club, a new job, a ball game, or wherever, and there she is: a stunningly beautiful woman at whom you can't stop staring. Whether blond or brunette, big-busted or athletic-looking, she has exactly the look that pushes all your buttons, that gets your heart racing and makes your pants feel tighter. What do you do?

Do you say to yourself, "I'm just an average joe, maybe a geeky one, and I'd stand no chance with her"—and then spend the rest of the day or evening dreaming about looking like someone else and making love to her? Or do you make a move, and if so, how do you fare? Do you walk out of there with her phone number—or better yet, her arm in yours—or do you drown your embarrassment in booze, wishing you could get such a woman?

The fame of a Hollywood star or the money of a wealthy entrepreneur are good enough to attract a hot woman. But most men are not so fortunate; for the 99 percent of you who are in that category, this book is designed to provide the help to realize your dreams.

You Can Do It

The techniques discussed here will work with any woman. You may want to practice them on average- or below-average-looking women to start with, just to prove to yourself that they work and that you can make them work. However, the goal here is to enable you to be successful with the very hottest, best-looking women because, let's face it: men rate a woman's looks as the most important, or nearly the most important, factor that makes a woman desirable, either as a bed partner or as a mate. So if you want the best for yourself, you naturally want a woman who is regarded as beautiful. And take it from me, Penthouse Pet of the Year and Ph.D. in psychology, you can do it. You *can* score with women who rate 8, 9, or even 10 on the beauty scale, with models, centerfolds, cheerleaders, sexy nurses, or that hot blonde in accounts payable.

I know that some of you might think that centerfolds only hook up with rock or movie stars, or at least jocks or rich businessmen who can ply them with diamonds and cars. And, yes, some of them do. Fame and fortune attract beautiful women like moths to a candle flame; like such moths, however, many centerfold models and the like burn out their youth and beauty on drug-addicted Hollywood wannabes. But, believe it or not, most don't. There are literally thousands of hot women who don't end up in the arms of those Playboy Mansion habitués, or who try that route and find it unsatisfying. Indeed, there are hundreds of super-sexy women who have fallen in love with, and married, average-looking guys with average-income jobs; and there are hundreds more who have slept with them. For each hot model who marries a rock star or billionaire, there are probably a dozen whose boyfriends or husbands are virtual unknowns with typical middle-class occupations. I know models who have spurned movie stars to marry UPS delivery men or auto mechanics—men who look nothing like a movie star or a typical sports hero. So never count yourself out in the game of romancing or scoring with beautiful women.

However, that is not to say that gorgeous women will necessarily fall for any "Joe Blow" from East Paducah. These women get approached, hit upon, propositioned, and even stalked by many men; they learn to be wary and skeptical of the average guy. You need to have something "special" that makes you stand out from the crowd, a combination of the right features, attitudes, and techniques that makes you attractive to a woman who knows she has many choices. It doesn't take magic, massive plastic surgery, or a million dollars to create that "special" image, but it does take work, effort, and some courage. That "something special" is what this book is all about.

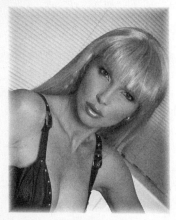

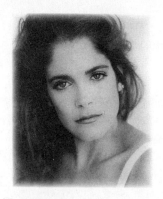

Penthouse model and Dr. Z's sister, Tatiana Z, has "learned through experience that the heart and brain of a man are far more important than his looks, status, or money. As for the physical attraction, it is his lips, eyes, and hands that draw my attention."

Playboy's Miss December 1982 Charlotte Kemp has dated NFL football players, NHL hockey players, Formula One race car drivers, rock stars and other musicians, actors, and PGA golf players, as well as regular guys and moguls.

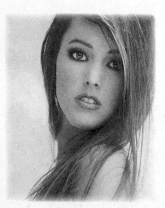

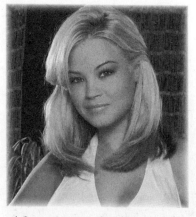

January 2007 Pet of the Month Erica Ellyson says, "I'm not too good to talk to anyone or date anyone, no matter who they are or what they do. Everyone deserves a deeper look and is interesting in their own ways."

November 2006 Pet of the Month Brea Lynn confesses her love for uniforms: "My boyfriend wears a uniform to work and I love it when he comes home for lunch in it!"

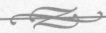

PART 1

The Art of Picking Up

Hot Babes

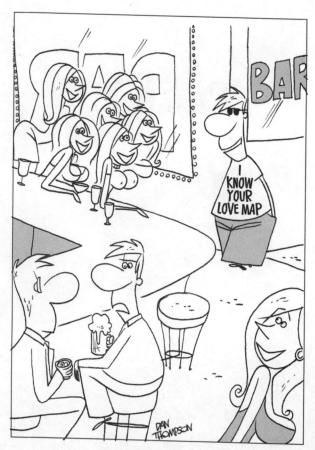

"Great, now we don't have a chance with
these women!"

One

Prototypes and Love Maps: Being the Lid for Her Pot

Love Maps, Prototypes, and Childhood Crushes

Women think men are led around by their penises. We're not. It points us in a direction, I'll give you that.

—Garry Shandling

It is a stroke of good fortune to find one who is worth seducing. . . . Most people rush ahead, become engaged or do other stupid things, and in a turn of the hand everything is over, and they know neither what they have won nor what they have lost.

—Søren Kierkegaard, *The Seducer's Diary*

Do you wonder why you seem to be attracted to a particular type of woman, like tall and blond, while your best friend prefers petite brunettes with curly hair? Your preferences are dictated in large part by the "love map" that you formed in childhood, a mental blueprint that contains the key characteristics you believe describe your ideal mate. Oftentimes, these beliefs are subconscious; they may have formed when you were too small to even understand the concept of sexual attraction. But they dominate our choices in mates, whether for a one-night stand or for marriage, because it is the sight or presence of a person that triggers our pre-set love maps, which leads to the release of the hormones in our brains that in turn cause sexual arousal. Women form the same love maps, and their idea of who is attractive to them might work for or against you. You never know without giving it a shot.

▸ *All of us have love maps or prototypes that were formed in childhood and dictate whom we are attracted to.*

For example, when I was about seven, my tall, dark-haired older cousin from the countryside came to visit us in Kiev. I used to love to sit in his lap and gaze at his face. He was a marine, with a uniform with shiny buttons, Gypsy looks with wavy locks, and a wicked sense of humor—very irreverent toward authority. I thought he was just about the most handsome, interesting male in my family; and lo and behold, when I grew older, I found that I was always attracted to men who looked and acted like my cousin. If you are tall, dark-haired, freedom-loving, and have a wild sense of humor and an antiauthoritarian bent, I am likely to fall for you if given a chance.

Every woman has a different "map." Take Pamela Anderson as an example—her choice of Tommy Lee and Kid Rock clearly indicates that she likes tattooed and pierced rock musicians with a bad-boy side. To me, and to many of my model friends, Kid Rock is downright ugly, a total greasebag. But to Pammy, the guy looks totally different. Another centerfold I know must have "imprinted" early on a male with an underbite, because she has always found the jutting jawline to be attractive. Another model that I know has the prototype of an artistic bohemian as her love map, which has always drawn her to creative men with beards and long hair. Cecille Gahr, Hawaiian Tropic contest winner and the actress on the TV series *Beauty and the Geek,* admits that she has a thing for geeks and that she dated quite a few of them in her life. "I am talking about the glasses and the curly short hair," she confesses in an interview for *Steppin' Out* magazine. Other centerfolds, like Tera Patrick, have a thing for men who are dominant, who take charge of them and their careers. Penthouse Pet Natalia Cruze (Sophia Santi) only goes out with black or very dark-skinned men, even though she is Caucasian. And Suzanne, the radio host of WRAT, finds herself drawn to men with big noses, like Adrien Brody and Gerard Depardieu. The variety of men that turn hot women on is endless.

▶ *Knowing your own love map will help you become more confident in dating.*

This "love map" of what men and women want in a mate develops during critical periods in early and late childhood as a result of a child's exposure to various people, and it is based on experiences with particular adults whom the child finds attractive and pleasurable. The love map is then "imprinted" or "hard-wired" into our psyches and becomes the inner scorecard that we use to rate the suitability of potential mates. Most people feel intense passion and drive when they find a person that fits their deep-rooted childhood ideal. As Robert Greene notes it in his book *The Art of Seduction,* "When a person has such a deep effect on you it transforms all of your subsequent maneuvers. Your face and gestures become more animated. You have more energy . . . Good seducers choose targets that inspire them but they know how and when to restrain themselves."[1] Knowing this means two things: (1) you can use your love map to focus your scoring techniques on the women you will really take off on, and (2) if you strike out with a particular chick, you can easily write it off as you must not have been on her "map." Make a list of all the things that would make a "perfect" woman, as well as a list of all the things that would be "deal killers." Knowing what you want will give you the confidence to be choosy, to seek the right woman, and to get over rejection by deciding you can find someone who fits your list better.

If you are interested in a particular woman, you may want to find out what kind of men she has dated in the past in order to figure out her love map. If a hot woman you are interested in tends to date slender professionals with glasses, you can certainly increase your chances of capturing her heart if you lose weight, get a short haircut, and don a business suit and faux glasses. Or you can decide that such a change is not worth your time and effort and quickly move on to a better prospect. If you are diametrically opposite from her imprinted love map or ideal mate prototype, the hot woman with an ample mating budget is not going to be interested—so don't waste your time. What you want is a woman who fits your love map and whose love map will fit you.

▶ *Knowing her love map will help you figure out if you can fit the prototype she is drawn to.*

You might notice from talking to a woman or watching her in action that she seems drawn to a particular prototype. You can decide to "become" that prototype. But first decide if that style really suits you. Are you drawn to free-spirited women who love rock musicians? Are you willing to grow your hair long, get a few tattoos, and get involved in a rock band as a hobby? Or are you impressive discussing business affairs while dressed in a suit and tie? Then you should work on developing a serious professional look and target sexy women who would be attracted to that look. If you are drawn to women who are much younger than you, you need to maintain a youthful look and attitude and keep up with the latest pop-culture trends. If you love easygoing women with a good sense of humor, moonlight as a stand-up comedian. If you are attracted to the California girl prototype, there is no better way to check out and pick up tanned beach bunnies than by becoming a lifeguard. If you love slender fashion model types, take up photography as a hobby and attend fashion photography workshops (where models are usually hired to pose). Do you get turned on by fit, shapely women? Prepare to hit the gym yourself. As you will see in the section below, we tend to select partners based on similarity, so if you tend to prefer certain qualities in women, it is helpful to cultivate the same in yourself.

One prototype is a no-brainer. If your occupation calls for you to wear a uniform, capitalize on it. Almost all women, including the hottest ones, are attracted to men in uniform, particularly those that signify courage and virility. For example, many women find the firefighter prototype irresistible because it is associated with courage, risk-taking, and kindness (qualities that women find universally appealing, as we will discuss later). Kim Cattrall's character in HBO's *Sex and the City* admitted to being attracted to the firefighter prototype: "You fantasize about a man with a Park Avenue apartment and a nice big stock portfolio. . . . For me it's a fireman with a nice big hose." Playmate Charlotte Kemp had a firefighter boyfriend for three years: "I loved his compassion, leadership, and confidence."

Pet of the Year Julie Strain has always found firefighters to be extremely attractive. "Men in uniform are hot and they live their lives to protect the world. After 9/11, I go up to firefighters all the time and thank them for saving our lives," she says, getting teary-eyed. So if you have a risk-taking trait, consider becoming a volunteer firefighter.

Soldier and sailor uniforms also symbolize courage and strength. Similarly, if you are a police officer, you might find it easier to pick up women while wearing your police uniform and talking about your latest crime scene victories. I know several Playmates, such as Tylyn John, who ended up marrying police officers. Auto racing or motocross, or any signifier of a risk-taking profession or hobby, will also appeal to many sexy women, as they are often drawn to guys who are daredevils. Penthouse Pet Brea Lynn confesses her love for uniforms: "My boyfriend wears a uniform to work and I love it when he comes home for lunch in it!" Pet of the Year Jamie Lynn is definitely attracted to a bad-boy prototype: "I like a man with a bigger build and tattoos; however, no musicians. I do like men in prison blues, like the guys on prison break." Unlike Jamie Lynn, Pet of the Year Runner-up Krista Ayne likes musicians: "The rocker type always catches my eye first, although I have dated all different types. I am definitely a sucker for a Mohawk or really cool hair. Tattoos and piercings are really sexy, but not a must."

Personally, I have always been attracted to "men in white"—doctors, scientists, and laboratory researchers. One day I dislocated my shoulder, and I went to the emergency room to have it put back in place. The man who came to help me was tall and dark-haired, and he was wearing that white medical coat. He acted with a lot of confidence and authority, so I immediately assumed he was a physician and equally promptly concluded that he was hot. I eagerly gave him my cell phone number and looked forward to hooking up with him. However, when I finally did go out with him, I found out he was an X-ray technician; he got a free score on the "love map" look, uniform and attitude alone, though.

Pet of the Year Heather Vandeven also has a definite prototype. "I've always liked tall men who are a bit strange but extremely intelligent, such as Anthony Bourdain, Howard Stern, and Jeff Goldblum," she says. Pet of the Year Runner-up Courtney Taylor also likes intelligent men. She is also attracted to men who are athletic: "Cyclists are so hot in their tight shirts and shorts."

▶ *You can decide to fit one of the prototypes popular with women.*

Finally, what appeals to women with high dating budgets is distinctiveness, excellence, or notoriety—in any field. If you excel at your chosen profession or hobby to the point where you will become recognized and respected for whatever you do, you will have an easier time attracting sexy women. If you think this is too hard to do, just take my friend Timmy, for example. He became paralyzed from the neck down after a traffic accident. He had always loved beautiful women and refused to give up being around them after his paralysis. He opened his own modeling agency, Stars Models, out of his Manhattan apartment, specializing in glamour models. Although he had only partial use of one hand, he had a special phone installed and dedicated all of his time to calling potential clients and recruiting models. His dedication and drive paid off. His agency became known as the premier agency for booking swimsuit and lingerie models in New York. Now he is not only surrounded by beautiful women but he also ended up marrying one—an Asian woman who became attracted to his kindness and entrepreneurial spirit. She had always wanted to be a modeling scout herself, and by meeting Timmy she realized her dream of running her own modeling agency.

So pick a prototype that most suits your personality and work on projecting that image. Not only will it appeal to her subconscious idea of an ideal man but it will also give you a strong sense of self. The last thing a hot woman wants is a guy who vacillates about who he is or wants to be, who does not have strong opinions, convictions, or talents, or whose goal in life is partying or stamp collecting. Not having a defined self-image translates into not having a life—which means you are likely to make *her* your life. That smells of a potential stalker or control freak.

HOT WOMEN HANG-UPS

All women think they're ugly, even pretty women. . . . Even models and actresses, even the women you think are so beautiful that they have nothing to worry about do worry all the time. —ERICA JONG

Learning the love map of your desired woman is only half of what you need to know. Models and women who succeed or fail on their looks have hang-ups that are less common in ordinary, average-looking women. There are six hang-ups that generally apply to centerfold models or women of equivalent looks.

1. They are often very insecure. That's right, you heard me, very insecure. As pointed out by Erica Jong in the quote above, all women worry about their appearance—and beautiful women worry about their appearance far more than average ones! Surprising as it may seem, there is a sound psychological basis for this insecurity. Because our society puts a high value on physical beauty, girls who are born with good looks often grow up basing their entire self-esteem on their external appearance and fail to develop other sources of self-efficacy. Because beauty is fleeting and variable and, to some extent, depends on the eye of the beholder, such women often have a fluctuating self-esteem that requires a continuous validation of their desirability. Some achieve this by associating with handsome or high-status males, but others can be reassured by receiving continuous verbal validation of their lasting attractiveness. Understanding that you will be the vanity mirror to which she will turn to reaffirm her desirability is the key to dating a sexy woman. Whereas an average woman may put up with you admitting that other women are beautiful and even occasionally checking them out, a hot one will expect you to idolize her—and her alone—as "the fairest of them all."

2. They are often unhappy or neurotic. Although we often assume that beautiful people are happier than average ones, this is often not the case with beautiful women, particularly those who are in show business. Because beauties compete on the basis of their looks, something they have little control over, they often develop what psychologists call "external locus of control," a belief that they have little effect on their reality, a condition associated with depression. In addition, centerfolds and other models have undergone scrupulous scrutiny of magazine editors and modeling scouts, who are often very blunt and unkind in their criticism of imperfections (as some of you have seen in the TV show *The Agency*). They have been told over and over that they are too fat or too short or that their thighs are too wide or their breasts are not perky enough by the ultimate "arbiters of beauty"—editors and agents—and many of them internalize these beliefs as their own. Believe me, I was far happier with my face and body before I posed for *Playboy*, as the process of shooting a centerfold nearly destroyed my belief in my attractiveness. Every piece of clothing added to my body during my centerfold shoot was put there to cover some fatal flaw, some awful defect that was discussed by the photographers and editors right in front of me, as if I were a porcelain doll, not a live person with feelings.

Almost every centerfold I have met has had her face and body critically "dissected" by some modeling gatekeeper during the course of her career, and many have turned to plastic surgery to correct those flaws. As a result, models and actresses have a much higher incidence of psychological issues—depression, anxiety, eating disorders, borderline and histrionic personality disorders, substance abuse, and body dysmorphia—than average women do. For that reason, many men who date hot women become not only their lovers but also their de facto therapists. If you can understand the pain behind that gorgeous façade and not simply assume, like most men do, that beauty equals happiness, therein lies a pathway to her heart.

3. They want to be more than sex objects. Ironically, while hot women enjoy the power of their sex appeal, they detest when men treat them as mere sex objects. Although being "objectified" can feel flattering and empowering, particularly to average women who do not get sexual attention as often, it can also become burdensome, self-limiting, and stigmatizing. After all, our society views sex objects as dumb, self-absorbed, and existing solely to be used for sexual pleasure. Because beautiful women are more likely to have been victims of sexual abuse, sexual harassment, and nonconsensual sexual acts, they may also become more defensive about being viewed as a sexual object.

Thus, a majority of these women fall for men who appreciate them (or at least pretend to) for other aspects of their personality. In fact, both in my experience and according to surveys of beautiful women, one of the most desired compliments that you can give her is one that would emphasize positive characteristics above and beyond her looks. "You are not only beautiful, but very intelligent," "You have a great personality," "You are a joy to be around," "You are so down-to-earth despite your beauty"—these types of compliments are guaranteed to ingratiate you in her eyes. No matter how hot a woman is, she is unlikely to appreciate your "blond bimbo" jokes. The more you treat her as a person and not as an object of sexual gratification, the more likely she is to fall for you.

4. They are usually "high maintenance." Hot women go to great lengths to look hot. They improve their bodies with exercise and plastic surgery; their facial features with creams, injections, and cosmetics; their hair, nails, and lashes with color and extensions; and they spend a considerable amount of time choosing the right clothing that flatters their figures. While teenagers can look great with minimal makeup and no effort, when a woman hits her mid-twenties, age starts to take its toll. To retain her beauty, she will strive to purchase even more expensive accoutrements: designer clothes, makeup, and other beauty products. She is going to spend time and money in parlors and spas, in health clubs, and in other facilities that provide beautifying and age-delaying treatments. She might spend three times what an average-looking woman spends on these things, which means she has less to spend on other things, like food or entertainment. She needs a man who understands and supports her desire to remain at the top of the beauty totem pole, a man who indulges her love of clothes, shopping, and dressing up, and a man who is generous in providing her with the means both to stay beautiful and to show it off. You don't need mil-lions to make it with a model, but you can't be thinking of saving up for distant rainy days either. Beauty always comes at a price!

5. They often feel "entitled." Most beauties have an exaggerated set of expectations. A majority of hot women know the powerful effect their looks have on men, and they might expect "special treatment" from the world based on their belonging to an "elite" group of sex goddesses. This expectation might go well beyond what most men, or society in general, are willing to afford them, as beauty is not necessarily accompanied by brains, talents, or any special abilities that carry high economic rewards. Nevertheless, a sexy woman's expectation of special treatment, or "narcissistic entitlement" as psychologists call it, cannot be ignored. Instead, it must be pandered to—at least until she grows out of it—and used in your approach. As "princesses-in-waiting" who believe that they are entitled to that special kiss from their prince charming, such women will expect you to be the prince who will give them that symbolic kingdom. As we will see, when you get her into your bed, you can make this happen, but to get there, you will need to project yourself as a prince who is not intimidated by her royal highness.

6. They can afford to be picky. It's true that they expect "higher value" in men they select as lovers. The psychology of mate selec-tion suggests that men and women higher in overall desirability are more discriminating and impose higher standards in their mate selection preferences than do those lower in desirability. Evo-lutionary psychologist Norman Li has portrayed this mate selection preference in terms of the "budget[ed] allocation of mating dollars" that each person has. When a woman's mating budget is tight (that is, when a woman is only a 3 or 4 on a scale of desirability), she will go for guys who possess the bare "necessities," such as intel-ligence, work ethic, and a sense of humor. However, the women with larger "budgets" (the 9's and 10's), tend to require more qualities in a man, such as physical attractiveness, a high-paying job, noteworthy skills, or other qualifications. These women can afford to spend their "surplus" mating dollars on obtaining mates who are especially creative or who have interesting personalities.

This then is the target of your seduction: an often insecure, beauty-obsessed, depressed, picky narcissist who thinks she deserves to be a princess and doesn't like to be treated as a mere sex object, and who has her own unique love map of the man who, she imagines, will be her prince charming. It doesn't sound like the sort of woman you would bring home to Mama, yet she has the looks to knock your socks off, so you wouldn't pass her up for anyone or anything. Now, how are you going to land her?

TIP #1: Find your love map, which characterizes your ideal woman, figure out the prototype that she is drawn to, and adjust your own image (i.e., funny comedian, brave firefighter, ambitious businessman, etc.) accordingly. Then work on standing out among all the other guys that project a similar image. Keep in mind that hot women are insecure, neurotic, high-maintenance, picky, and feel entitled to special treatment but want to be appreciated for more than their looks, and be ready to deal with it and use it to your advantage. ✦

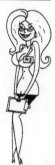

Top 12 Most Popular Prototypes to Emulate

The reasons why these prototypes are the most popular is that they evoke qualities that women are drawn to (as you will see in subsequent chapters).

1. The Rescuer (firefighter, lifeguard, doctor, paramedic, and other medical personnel). Many women, including yours truly, are attracted to "men in white." The minute a guy mentions he is a physician, especially a surgeon, he scores major points in my love book. And believe it or not, it has nothing to do with money; I dated one physician who was perpetually broke because he worked almost entirely on a pro bono basis with indigent populations. Firefighters are universally admired and adored by women.

2. The Defender (soldier, police officer, bodyguard). Many hot women are afraid of violence and want to feel safe, protected, and taken care of. They love a courageous, strong man who is respected and deferred to by the general population. I know quite a few hotties who married police officers, soldiers, and bodyguards.

3. The Athlete (bodybuilder, martial arts master, tennis player). As mentioned above, women are attracted to men with big guns. By working out on a regular basis, you will more than double your chances of scoring with hot women. If you love to hit the gym, consider becoming a part-time personal trainer, as hot women often hire them. Choosing to excel in a popular recreational sport such as golf or scuba diving will definitely add a point or two to your overall sex appeal.

4. The Musician (rock star, troubadour, composer, singer). Music has always been used to inspire romantic feelings and sexual desires. I vividly remember falling for one of my sister's exboyfriends as he serenaded her with ballads on his guitar, making both of us melt. If you have any musical talents, work on developing them. Sing her Carly Simon's hit "You're So Vain," and she is guaranteed to love you for it.

5. The Entertainer (joker, jester, comedian, clown, harlequin, pantomimist, ventriloquist, magician). Just like music and movement, laughter elevates her mood and makes her feel good. No wonder women are attracted to the guys who can tell a good joke or make a funny face. So if you hone your funny bone, you will increase your chances of scoring. Jenny McCarthy is not the only one who finds Jim Carrey's silly faces very sexy!

6. The Artist (painter, sculptor, photographer). Most beautiful women love to have their beauty immortalized and deified through art forms. If you have an artistic talent, you have a direct path into their heart (and their pants). My friend Jon Paul is a romance-novel cover illustrator. Needless to say, beautiful women are constantly contacting him about posing for his work. If you can't draw or sculpt, take photography lessons. In my experience, photographers have no problem scoring with sexy women (I have slept with a few myself!).

7. The Entrepreneur (businessman, attorney). Because hot women have a sense of entitlement, most of them are not keen on the idea of having to work for a living. And because modeling and show business do not offer a consistent income, they are attracted to men who have big business ideas.

8. The Good Samaritan (philanthropist, animal lover, child rights advocate). Empathy and compassion are very high on any woman's list of attributes she wants in a man. There is no greater way to endear a woman than by showing kindness toward an animal or a child.

9. The Intellectual (professor, commentator, MENSA member). Believe it or not, intelligence is a highly coveted quality by hot women. If you are a walking encyclopedia of facts and stats, use your knowledge to attract hot women. Just make sure the facts you recite are entertaining, and you don't come across as an intellectual snob.

10. The Psychic (palm reader, tarot card reader, astrologist, hypnotist, medical intuitive). Most women are very intuitive and are drawn to men who appear to possess greater than average male intuition. Pick some mystic new age philosophy and bone up on it: if you can talk about Kabbalah to her, she'll be all ears. A great test to see if she is into mysticism is to ask her, "Have you read or watched *The Celestine Prophecy*?" If she responds positively and enthusiastically, then tell her that you feel synchronicity with her and that you would like to uplift her with your energy (make sure to at least scan the book beforehand).

11. **The Writer** (poet, novelist, songwriter, scriptwriter, producer, director). Hot women love men who are facile with words—they love to be admired and immortalized in any art form, and who can sing their laurels better than eloquent men?

12. **The Agent** (attorney, book agent, modeling or acting scout). The agent has an obvious appeal to hot women because many of them seek fame and fortune in show business. The agent holds the magic key to that highly coveted world of glory and recognition.

Two

Teeth and Pecs:
Putting Your Best Foot Forward

FIRST GLANCE IS THE DECISIVE ONE

Let's face it, a date is like a job interview that lasts all night. The only difference between the two is that there are very few job interviews where there's a chance you will end up naked at the end of it.   —JERRY SEINFELD

Indeed, dating is very similar to interviewing for a job. To get a low-paying manual job, you do not need much in terms of qualifications. The same might be said for meeting and dating a below-average-looking woman. However, before you can get a prestigious, well-paying job, you need to develop the appropriate qualifications—presentable appearance, academic degrees, work experience, and social skills—to come across well during an interview. Psychologists call this "impression management," and meeting and dating beautiful women require the same kind of impression management. Remember that you will be competing with many other applicants for her attention and interest, so the bare qualifications are not sufficient here.

While good looks are not a prerequisite to dating a sexy model—indeed, some of my centerfold girlfriends are married to men I think are downright ugly—you cannot ignore the fact that what you look like is the first thing she will notice. The old adage "You never get a second chance to make a first impression" is all too true. The people we meet form up to 90 percent of their opinions about us in the first several minutes, and our physical desirability is usually assessed in the first ten seconds! What is worse, social research indicates that the initial impressions we make on others tend to persist. Moreover, such impressions are quite resistant, even in the face of later contradictory information. To see your own propensity for making quick first impressions, read the description of the two hypothetical persons below and try to picture their personalities:

Person 1:
    intelligent, industrious, impulsive, critical, stubborn, envious

Person 2:
    envious, stubborn, critical, impulsive, industrious, intelligent

Which one have you found to be more likeable? The majority of people report more favorable reactions to the first person, even though the two lists of traits are identical in content, differing only in sequence.[2] Those who were exposed to the first list of traits reported the imaginary person as more sociable, humorous, and happy than those in the second group.[3] Once we draw a conclusion about a person, we tend to interpret the rest of his or her behavior in light of that information.

▸ *First impressions are lasting ones, and your appearance matters.*

For example, my first husband met me for the first time in a limousine. He was dressed in an Armani suit, designer sunglasses, with a dark tan, an Italian leather briefcase, and a Cuban cigar in hand. He was the epitome of cool, at least to me at the time, and I persisted in imagining that he was a successful criminal defense attorney with style and savoir faire. Only after a few years of marriage did I realize that he was really a lying sleazebag. But I wasn't the only one who fell for his schtick: he'd had two wives and many very attractive girlfriends before me, and after I divorced him, he scored with two more rich, elegant women who supported his habits. So first impressions are BIG, and you will want to make them the best.

How does this fact translate into the dating scene? Your appearance and demeanor will be the first thing the women you meet will use to decide whether or not you get a chance to score; indeed, they will draw conclusions about what you are like before you even open your mouth! A majority of the centerfolds I interviewed said they make up their mind about whether they want to date a guy "within the first ten minutes." So before you step out to pick up that super-sexy babe, you need to pay attention to your appearance. By that I don't mean running out and getting an extreme makeover. A man who devotes too much attention to enhancing his appearance can hurt his competitive chances by appearing homosexual or narcissistic[4]—just think of George Hamilton's parody of good looks, with his nose job and perpetually overly tanned face. But slight modifications to your grooming and dress habits can make a huge difference to that first impression your dream girl will form about you!

BEING THE PRIME CUT IN THE MEAT MARKET

Men ought to be more conscious of their bodies as an object of sexual desire.   —GERMAINE GREER

Although women are less likely than men to evaluate prospective mates based on their looks, women do pay attention to a guy's overall appearance during their mate selection process. The typical social settings for matchmaking—clubs, parties, organization meetings, etc.—are meat markets for women, and they will size up the beef based on its overall state of health, coloring, and wrapping. Obviously, there is a wide variability in what women may find attractive in a male, based on her ideal mate prototype, and there are some characteristics that are intractable (such as height). But there are several general characteristics that all women find desirable in a guy: good grooming, dental hygiene, and weight control. Most centerfolds I interviewed marked "yellow or missing teeth" and "obviously overweight" as instant turnoffs. These factors are universally important because they reflect a man's state of health, and women worldwide prefer men who are healthy.[5] Guess what? You can control these factors to make your first impression a robust, healthy one.

Why is health such a turn-on to women? Evolutionary psychologists argue that women have developed a preference for healthy-looking males over centuries of natural selection. Even among the brutish Neanderthals, an unhealthy male would have been less likely to provide for the woman and their children, and if he'd had a risk of dying young, she could have gotten stuck with all the kids by herself. Moreover, if she'd thought his health problems would affect their children, he would not have rated highly on her primitive Match.com list. Thus, women might have developed an innate, subconscious preference for healthy males.[6]

Of course, you men are the same way. All those attributes of feminine beauty that you desire—clear skin, big boobs, bubble butt, and long silky hair—are signs of health and youth in a woman, as well as an ability to bear healthy children. We are all products of our biological sex drives, which in turn are tied to our evolutionary need to reproduce. Before there was language, there were looks; and we have inherited that instinct for spotting the prime cuts.

But it doesn't matter whether you are actually in perfect health or not as long as you *appear* healthy. It's a little like fake breasts:

most guys like breasts whether they are real or silicone if their size fits their love map and they look healthy. The same goes for hair extensions and fake eyelashes. It's the appearance that counts. So it is for women too. What are the signs of good health that women look for in men? The most obvious ones are clear skin that is not broken out, dull, or pale; bright eyes; shiny hair; a full set of white teeth; healthy-looking nails; a normal weight range, and a good smell.

▶ *Women prefer guys that look healthy, and good bodily and dental hygiene are signifiers of good health.*

Needless to say, good oral hygiene and grooming habits cannot be understated. Two of the most frequently listed turnoffs on data sheets of Playboy centerfolds are "bad breath" and "body odor," both of which can be easily corrected with good dental and physical hygiene. If regular dental care doesn't take care of your bad breath, you might be genetically predisposed to halitosis—constant bad breath caused by an excessive amount of plaque that adheres to the whole mouth. This can be fixed by a series of deep-cleaning treatments by a dentist. And try to avoid alcohol-based mouthwash, which can dry out the mouth. Use an alcohol-free one instead. If deep dental cleaning doesn't improve your breath, you might have a stomach bacteria called *H. pylori*, which causes bad breath but can be easily eliminated by a course of antibiotics. If you are a smoker and a coffee drinker, you need to be particularly mindful of your breath, and it's probably a good idea to bleach your teeth as well, as they tend to get yellow from the nicotine and caffeine. The easiest and costliest way to get your teeth pearly white is by going to a cosmetic dentist, but if you don't want to spend the money, pick up a cheap bleaching kit at the local pharmacy.

If you think that the shade of your teeth should not matter in attracting a woman, you are deeply mistaken. In a recent survey, women were asked to identify one thing that they look for in a man. Three-quarters responded that pearly whites are a key to attraction.[7] And in my survey of Penthouse Pets, almost every one indicated that bad teeth are a major turnoff. Pet of the Year Julie Strain stressed the importance of good dental hygiene: "Please brush and floss regularly—I don't want to see plaque on your teeth!" Yellow, unkempt teeth are associated with aging, disease, decay, drug use, and lower socioeconomic status. And while many women can overlook a beer gut or hairy ears, no hot woman likes a guy whose smile looks like a jack-o'-lantern's. Smiles are the most important factor in human interaction and, particularly, attraction. And since a kiss is going to be your entrée to getting laid with this babe, you should want to make your mouth as inviting as possible for kisses!

▶ *If you can change only one thing about your appearance, improve the look of your teeth.*

Taking regular showers and using deodorants should be sufficient to keep your body smelling fresh and odor-free. A fresh smell of sweat (as if you just finished playing tennis) is actually a turn-on for most women, as it contains pheromones, the odorless chemicals that serve to attract the opposite sex. It's when your sweat is broken down by the bacteria on your skin over time that it acquires an unpleasant odor. For that reason, don't overdo the colognes—they mask these natural pheromones that your body emits, which turn women on.

As Penthouse Pet Melissa Jacobs put it: "It's one thing to smell good, but it's another thing to smell like the cologne section of the department store. Spray the body a little bit, or spray it into the air and walk through the mist." If you are prone to excessive sweating, consider getting Botox injections in your armpits.

When you do use cologne, choose one with ingredients that mimic natural pheromones. Research has confirmed that women are more attracted to men who wear pheromone-based colognes (or pheromone-based aftershave additives, such as 10X).[8] In addition, these substances may enhance the wearer's feelings of attractiveness and self-assurance. Besides pheromones, certain scents may also be appealing to women: studies have found that women have an acute ability to smell musk,[9] a compound that is similar to the hormone testosterone, and is used in many colognes. Another study reported that women are attracted to a black licorice scent. So, be sure to pick up licorice or Good 'n Plenty and keep it in your shirt pocket, or order Sambuca or a shot of Jägermeister before heading over to talk to her.

▸ *Use pheromone additives in colognes and aftershaves to subliminally increase your attractiveness to women.*

As with dental hygiene, guys often ignore their skin—and although wrinkles look virile on most men, and nobody notices an occasional pimple, cystic acne gives a man a decidedly "juvenile" look, which is a turnoff to most women. There are a number of over-the-counter and prescription medicines for treating cystic acne, including the most powerful one—Accutane. In addition, there are lasers and other treatments. So take care of those pustulent pimples before hitting the dating scene! In addition, if you spend most of your time indoors and your skin tends to look pale, you might want to hit the tanning salon from time to time or opt for the healthier alternative, a fake spray tan. A light hint of color is definitely perceived as attractive. In one study, pallor of the skin, open sores, and lesions were immediately perceived as signs of ill health and were universally regarded as unattractive.[10]

Guys often get insecure about their height. However, most models I have interviewed did not rate a guy's height as very important. Although Pet of the Year Julie Strain is 6'1", she admits she "has dated guys 5'6" because their hearts made up for their height."

Many men also feel insecure about their hair, particularly if they are prone to male pattern baldness. However, "a full head of hair" was not one of the characteristics that most centerfolds marked as important on my questionnaire. My advice—don't try to disguise your bald spots by combing them over or doing some other maneuvers! And unless you can afford a top-of-the-line plastic surgeon, do not go for cheap hair plugs. Instead, keep your hair short or shave it off. Baldness can be quite sexy—just think of Bruce Willis and Andre Agassi. While some women find some facial and body hair to be a turn-on, most women are turned off by visible hair where it isn't attractive—such as the ears and nose. This may be an evolutionary preference—as men evolved, they shed most of their body hair. In fact, the trend with young women is to prefer men with less body hair. Because of this, many men are turning to permanent hair removal with laser technology (which is almost painless). So if your back looks like a Neanderthal's, you might want to consider modern technology to improve your chances with hot women. Many men are also grooming their pubic hair to make their genitals appear larger and more inviting for oral sex (more about that in Part 3).

▶ *Manicured male hands are in, raggedy nails are out.*

Finally, when grooming yourself, do not forget about your extremities. A woman will often look at a guy's hands to determine his health and professional status. If you have a nail fungus, get it treated by a dermatologist. Although chapped male hands will probably not break the deal, women are often turned off by dirty, raggedy nails (if you don't believe me, just check out the centerfold preferences table in the back). So make sure to clean and file them on a regular basis, or better yet, get a regular manicure and pedicure. If the thought of putting clear nail polish on your nails nauseates you, just ask the nail technician to cut, file, and buff your nails. By the way, nail salons provide an excellent opportunity to meet women, because generally women are feeling happy and relaxed when getting pampered, and a positive emotional state is a prerequisite to a successful first impression (as you will see in the following chapter). Plus, sitting in the chair for long periods is pretty boring, and I know for myself that if a guy was in the next chair, I would certainly be receptive to a conversation. Finally, many manicurists and cosmetologists are quite cute, so even if the other customers don't float your boat, you can always pick up the girl playing with your toes.

You can also improve your overall appearance through physical exercise. One study of body types found that people's perceptions of strangers' personalities were strongly influenced by their physiques. Overweight individuals were perceived less favorably than thin or muscular individuals. Thin individuals were perceived as intelligent but fearful, and muscular individuals were most likely to be perceived as being healthy, brave, and good-looking. While your favorite hottie might have brainy wimps in her love map, chances are she is going to be more attracted to the jock types with the muscles. The fact that society rewards athletes with fame and fortune tends to reinforce the jock as the alpha male in women's eyes, so it's no wonder that the musclemen have the edge.

My sister, who is both a model and an archaeologist, is typical of this type. You can be any age, race, nationality, or level of handsomeness, but you won't get a second look from Tat unless you have some bulge in your biceps. Of course, Tat is also an ultra-buff martial arts aficionado and likes to spend her summers hiking up mountains in Peru looking for lost civilizations, so it's somewhat natural that she would fall for athletic builds. I, on the other hand, can leave the muscle-bound in the gym and go out with the brainy guy (so long as he is tall and dark haired), but as models go, I am in the distinct minority. Most of the Playboy and Penthouse centerfolds I know grew up in towns where the jocks were the local heroes, so the odds are high that building up some muscle tone will increase your desirability to the most attractive women.

In fact, while a man's attraction to a woman is strongly influenced by her face, women are more likely to be attracted to a guy's body. Indeed, one survey of women's sexual preferences revealed that broad shoulders, muscular arms, a small butt, narrow hips, and a flat belly are among the top ten physical characteristics that women find to be sexually appealing.[11] Facial features didn't make the top ten at all. Instead, women thought that displays of strength (even such relatively mundane ones such as opening a jar or lifting a chair) were very sexy; and that bigger displays of athleticism (like flexing muscles, playing sports, boasting about athletic prowess, etc.) would make a man especially attractive.[12] Note that while being an athlete will probably get you a date with most hotties, you don't have to be David Beckham to score. Any guy can open a jar, and that is enough muscle for most women. So you don't have to look like Arnold Schwarzenegger (in his prime) to attract your favorite centerfold. Regular exercise will help you shed extra pounds and develop enough muscle tone to approximate the mesomorph physique that most women find desirable.

Moreover, in addition to losing weight and gaining muscle tone, working out makes you feel happier by flooding your brain with endorphins, the feel-good hormones. It also increases testosterone levels in your body, which has a positive impact on your mood and overall well-being. Testosterone is a masculinizing hormone responsible for your muscle mass, deep, manly voice, and sexual desire—all qualities that women find attractive. You can boost your testosterone levels with as little as 40 minutes of weight lifting twice a week. Testosterone increases the most with short, intense bursts of physical activity, while it decreases with prolonged activity, especially frequent endurance training. Fitness also leads to better posture through improved muscle coordination (posture is one of the first things women notice) and an increase in strength, flexibility, and stamina (which is a definite benefit for sexual performance). Exercise also improves cardiovascular health, which has a direct correlation with sexual function. Regular exercise actually strengthens the heart, resulting in more blood and oxygen flow throughout the body, including your genital area. Yes, guys, the best way to maintain those rock-hard teenage erections is by engaging in regular physical exercise! A majority of erectile dysfunction is related to endothelial dysfunction (thickening of the blood vessel lining due to heart disease), which is preventable with regular exercise and a healthy diet. Though the symptoms of heart disease may not surface until middle age, the onset of disease can start taking place as early as the teens. Exercising for twenty to thirty minutes three times a week can reverse years of cardio neglect, thus preserving your erectile function!

▸ *Working out will make you healthier, sexier, smarter, and better in the sack, and it will expose you to more sexy women, so do it!*

Because exercise increases blood and oxygen flow throughout the body, including the brain, it might make you smarter and faster on your feet—which definitely boosts your pickup skills! Studies have shown that those who exercise react more quickly to stimuli than their less fit counterparts, pointing to a possible link between motor and intellectual skills.

Finally, a fitness regimen also offers many psychological benefits, such as improved self-image and self-confidence. Athletes often recount the first time they surpassed what they believed to have been the limit of their skills and how this affected their opinions of themselves. Many of those who exercise report experiencing the "flow," a psychological feeling of being fully immersed in an activity that is at once demanding and rewarding, and which is considered one of the most enjoyable and valuable experiences a person can have.[13]

And don't forget an important side benefit to hitting the gym—it provides an opportunity to meet sexy, fit women!

TIP #2: Enhance your appearance with good grooming (yes, tweeze those nose hairs), good dental hygiene (bleach those teeth and brush your tongue), attention to your skin and nails, and physical exercise. The single most important part of your appearance is your smile, so invest in improving your teeth if you need to. Choose colognes and aftershaves with pheromone additives, and indulge in some black licorice, as it attracts women. ✦

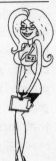

Top 10 Worst Physical Turnoffs in a Guy

Wondering why you haven't gotten many dates lately? All you may need is a quick physical makeover. Here's Dr. Z's critical eye for a straight guy:

1. Cystic acne. Everyone gets a pimple or two here and there, but if you are covered with those pustulent red volcanoes, go—run—to your dermatologist. A few months of Accutane, and you will be prime dating material again.

2. Raggedy nails. Women love manly hands, but if your nails look like jagged saws with suspicious black fungus underneath, she is unlikely to yearn for your touch. File and clean them regularly, or get a manicure, even if you think it's gay. And unless you plan on keeping your socks on (which I strongly advise against), you might get a pedicure, too.

3. Flatulence and belching. You might have been the star of your class in burping contests, but keep that achievement to yourself. Eat slower, chew your food well, cut down on sodas, and take frequent bathroom breaks if you can't control your gaseous outbursts.

4. Missing teeth. We all lose our teeth eventually, but if yours are leaving you at your prime dating age, run to your dentist. Missing teeth are not only aesthetically displeasing, they are often a sign of drug abuse or gum disease, which is implicated in the development of impotency. For all those reasons, women are evolutionarily programmed to dislike toothless men. And while you are getting your incisors back, you might as well have your teeth bleached, especially if you are a smoker.

5. Body odor. A fresh scent of male perspiration can actually be a turn-on to women, as it contains pheromones. But if you reek of stale sweat, she will run from you as fast as she can. If you tend to sweat bullets, do not try to mask your sweat with cologne, as that makes a particularly onerous odor, but use a strong deodorant or get a shot of Botox under your arms.

6. Bad breath. Nothing kills a kissing mood quicker than bad breath. All of us are prone to stinky mouth from time to time, so get some of those Listerine breath strips, or chew on a lemon or orange peel. Brushing your tongue regularly also helps kill stench-causing bacteria. But if your bad breath is strong and persistent, you are probably suffering from stomach bacteria called *H. pylori*, for which you need to take a course of antibiotics.

7. Hirsute nostrils. Unless it's on your head, hair is not in vogue lately. If you tend to grow hairs in your nose or ears, pluck them regularly, or get them lasered out.

8. Man boobs. Most women don't mind a spare tire around your waist, and even a little gut can be endearing. But if you are sporting male mammaries that compete in size with hers, you are probably suffering from a male condition called gynecomastia. With some simple surgery, your man boobs will be gone!

9. Goofy glasses. Unless Austin Powers is her idol, she will not appreciate your 1940s trifocals. Get some cool glasses, contacts, or Lasik.

10. Hair blunders. Unless you are a professional hairdresser, avoid cutting or coloring your own hair. Avoid teasing it unless you want to look like Donald Trump.

Three

Voice and Clothes: Croaking and Peacocking

TUNING YOUR MATING CALL

A good voice involves more than a high decibel level. . . . A voice without undue inflection may charm, soothe, calm, or arouse. A voice can also repel, infuriate, or actually make a listener ill.

—JOHNNY OLSON

The voice collects and translates your bad physical health, your emotional worries, your personal troubles.

—PLACIDO DOMINGO

Frogs croak, crickets chirp, cats howl, cows below—all over the animal kingdom, the male with the best roar scores. Indeed, the sexier a man's voice is, the more irresistible he is to a lot of women. A great example of this phenomenon is Howard Stern. Far from a classically handsome man, Howard has a deep, hypnotizing voice that many women (including me) find extremely alluring. Virtually every centerfold I have interviewed found Stern's voice and way of conversing to be a turn-on. And not surprisingly, one study found that men whose voices were rated most attractive by women had the most sex partners.

▸ *One of my theories is that men love with their eyes; women love with their ears.* —ZSA ZSA GABOR

When you speak, a woman attends more to your grammar, accent, and pitch than the content of what you are saying. A deep, masculine voice most appeals to women. High-pitched, tense voices that lack clarity are particularly unattractive because they come across as childish. We tend to perceive people with childlike voices to be weak and incompetent. I can personally attest to being turned off by such voices. In fact, I even rejected one extremely attractive lover—a good-looking and well-dressed physician who otherwise would have fit perfectly in my love map—because of his habit of leaving the longest messages on my voice mail in the most whiney, high-pitched voice imaginable. A guy who sounds like Mickey Mouse just can't pass himself off as a sex symbol, at least not to me or most models I know.

▸ *All really great lovers are articulate, and verbal seduction is the surest road to actual seduction.* —MARYA MANNES

Although not many guys have radio announcer voices, very few people have bad voices. Most of you can easily improve your voice by practicing a few simple rules. Here are some quick tips to help you improve the sound of your voice.

Deep breathing. A good voice has a lot of air power, which comes from deep breathing. Most people, however, take shallow breaths, filling their lungs only to a small percentage of their capacity. An air-deprived voice sounds monotone, and the ends of statements fade. Moreover, people who speak with a shallow voice often speak too fast, suggesting nervousness. To add power and sexiness to your voice, you need to make sure you are breathing from the diaphragm.

Place your hand on your diaphragm. Take in a deep breath and notice whether your diaphragm is moving. To heighten your awareness of how diaphragmatic breathing feels, raise your arms above your head or lie prone on a bed. The only way you will be able to breathe in these positions is from the diaphragm. Fantasize about a conversation with a girl that interests you while practicing that deep diaphragm-moving voice. Soon it might become second nature.

Watch your pitch. Begin paying attention to the fluctuations in the pitch of your voice. Try singing, but do it an octave lower on all your favorite songs. This exercise can help lower the voice. Also, when people get nervous, they tend to speak faster and their pitch tends to go up. So be particularly mindful of your pitch when you feel stressed or anxious. When you do feel nervous, slow down and deliberately pause between sentences. That deliberate pausing will dramatically improve your speech. Aim for a one- or two-second pause at the end of a statement or thought. Pausing should also help you eliminate nonwords such as "um" or "ah," which make a person sound unsure. And it will give you time to formulate your thoughts to make more compelling statements. However, be careful not to slow down to the point where people begin to finish your sentences just to help you finish.

Posture makes perfect. In addition to being mindful of pausing and breathing, pay attention to your posture. When you are slumping, your lungs are constricted, and they cannot move properly. Gesturing will also bring more air into your lungs, and your voice will sound more enthusiastic. Italian men have a habit of being very expressive with their hands when they talk; that may be a secret to their sexiness. So have a few imaginary conversations with your dream girl in front of a mirror so that you can get your hands and fingers into play as you talk.

Wet your whistle. If you tend to get dry mouth when you are nervous, drink lots of water or chew some gum beforehand. Avoid caffeinated drinks, which pull moisture from your throat. Likewise, stay away from milk products, because they tend to cause too much mucus in your mouth, and you will constantly be clearing your throat. Yup, that means no cappuccino lattes for you before you go out on a dating prowl!

Enunciate, enunciate, enunciate! Finally, and most important, make sure to enunciate your words properly. A guy who mumbles sounds dumb and uninteresting to women, and most won't make the effort to understand him. Mumbling is also a sign of nervousness or lack of self-confidence, which, as we will see, is a big turnoff to women. In addition to speaking clearly, animate your voice to avoid speaking monotonously. Words have color, enthusiasm, and even passion when spoken in a clear, animated voice. Think of JFK and the way he delivered his famous lines "Ask not what your country can do for you. . . ." There was a reason hot women like Marilyn Monroe thought he was sexy; it was not just his wavy hair or his money!

Put in some practice time. You can't train your voice to be a sexy one without practicing. Singers and public speakers spend many hours and days developing their voices, so you should not begrudge yourself the time to improve yours. One good way to practice, in addition to the suggestions above, is to buy a printed book and its audio version (making sure the audio reader has a deep male voice). Then record your voice reading from the book and listen to the tape, comparing it to the professional audio version. Work on trying to match the pitch, pacing, and enunciation of the professional reader. Another way is to listen to news broadcasters or commentators and to try to match their styles. If, after practicing, you still find yourself stumbling or mumbling, speaking in a high pitch, or if your accent is too heavy, get a voice coach.

Another way to improve your speaking skills is to take an acting class—it's also a great way to meet hot actress-wannabes!

TIP #3: To make your voice more attractive to women, lower your pitch, enunciate, slow down, and animate your voice. If you don't like how you sound, get a voice coach. ✦

Tip from the Scoring Experts *Gabriele D'Anunzio was a poet, novelist, and early-twentieth-century Italian fascist who won the attentions of actresses and noblewomen with ardent flattery and poetic words. Short, stocky, and grotesquely ugly, he hypnotized women with his soft, low voice. He spoke in alliterative phrases, flowery epithets, and suggestive images, articulating every word. Called "decadent" and a "perverter of public morals" by his critics, he preyed on women's insecurities by finding the most extravagant ways to praise them, using lilting language to tantalize their minds while he was moving in on their bodies.*

PROBLEM	SOLUTION
High pitch	Pause and lower
Mumbling	Enunciate every syllable
Nervousness	Slow down
Dry mouth	Drink water, avoid coffee
Monotone	Breathe deep
Hoarseness	Throat lozenges

PREENING YOUR FEATHERS

Seldom do people discern / Eloquence under a threadbare cloak.   —JUVENAL

Clothes make the man. Naked people have little or no influence on society.   —MARK TWAIN

Know, first, who you are; and then adorn yourself accordingly.   —EPICTETUS

One should either be a work of art, or wear a work of art.   —OSCAR WILDE

Do you ever wonder why male peacocks have those fancy tails, making them easy targets for predators? Darwin figured it out: to impress peahens.

Guys, as much as you hate to hear it, clothes are important! While clothes may not, in this day and age, "make the man," they may well enable the man to make the woman! Research consistently shows that what a guy wears is crucial to a woman's first impression; while men are more likely to be captivated by a woman's body and face, women are more likely to judge a man by his clothing. In one study, researchers showed men and women pictures of the opposite sex: some people in the photos wore chic designer outfits, whereas others wore cheaper and tackier clothes.[14] The women were asked a number of questions about the desirability of the men in the pictures as potential partners, ranging from "Whom would you choose to marry?" to "Whom would you choose for a one-night stand?" Women's answers to these questions correlated highly with the type of clothing the men in the photos wore—women consistently chose better-dressed men for both short-term and long-term interactions.[15] In another study, women who were shown slides of different men admitted to being more attracted to men who were wearing expensive clothing, such as three-piece suits, sports jackets, and designer jeans, than to men who were wearing cheap clothing, such as tank tops and T-shirts. The status and expense of a man's clothing had a strong effect on whether a woman was willing to have any type of involvement with him—from merely having coffee to accepting a marriage proposal. Men were photographed wearing a Burger King uniform with a blue baseball cap and a polo-type shirt. The same men were then photographed wearing a white dress shirt with a designer tie, a navy blazer, and a Rolex watch. After looking at the photographs, many women stated that they were unwilling to date, have sex with, or marry the men in the low-status costumes but were willing to consider all of the men in high-status garb.

Guys are always incredulous when I tell them about these studies. The reason men have a hard time believing that their choice of clothing is this important to women is that men pay little or no attention to how expensive a woman's outfit is (it could be from K-Mart but it's fine with him as long as it looks sexy on her). This gender difference is due to the fact that, subconsciously, a woman is far more concerned about a guy's economic status than a man is about a woman's. Even though most women are more than capable of providing for themselves, thousands of years of evolution have programmed the female brain to attend to symbols of wealth in a man, which signifies his ability to provide for her offspring. Even if a woman is wealthy herself or only considering a one-night stand, her mind is subconsciously evaluating a guy as a potential provider for their potential offspring. So dress to impress and fool her evolutionarily programmed brain into being attracted to you! Footwear is also extremely important when it comes to impressing a hottie. All women adore shoes, and hot women are particularly partial to expensive footwear. You don't have to have Imelda Marcus's passion for shoes but you should invest in a pair or two of fine Italian shoes. "I always notice a guy's shoes, and if a guy is wearing dirty, beat-up Nikes, there is a high chance I won't talk to him," says Pet of the Month Brea Lynn.

▶ *Dress stylishly and/or in accordance with your prototype.*

Similarly, the color of the clothing you choose might influence her perception of you. Social psychologists who investigated the effect of clothing color on human perception concluded that people wearing black clothes are more likely to be judged as aggressive or masculine. When subjects were asked to rate professional football and hockey uniforms, teams wearing pants and jerseys that were at least 50 percent black were rated as bad, mean, and aggressive. Why do you think the Oakland Raiders are always known as a mean and dirty team—even though they aren't that way on the field?

Further studies found that clothing affects not only the perceptions of others but also the behavior of the person wearing it! In one famous experiment, groups of men were given different colored uniforms to wear while engaging in a series of athletic activities. Amazingly, the participants became more aggressive after only a few minutes of being clothed in black uniforms. Black is the color of pirates and other notorious tough guys, from Zorro to Dracula to today's wrestling heroes. Black is also stylish and timeless and makes people appear thinner. White is a sign of gentleness, purity, peace, and neutrality. People tend to think that men in white, like doctors and ice cream vendors are clean, kindly, friendly, and helpful. So the old dichotomy between black-hatted bad guys and white-hatted good guys has its impact on the dating scene as well. When you are not sure what to wear, go with a white shirt. A pair of white linen pants is great for a summer day, as white is the perfect warm-weather color. But white shows dirt easily, so if you tend to be a bit of a klutz or slob, this is not the color for you. Also, if you are very blond or have a very light complexion, you may look washed out in white. White is a great choice for guys of Mediterranean descent. I personally love the clean, relaxed look of a dark-haired, tanned or dark-skinned man in a white linen shirt, blue jeans, and loafers on a summer day. He is the stranger who frequently appears in my sex-on-the-beach fantasies!

How does this apply to your choice of clothing? If you tend to be perceived as a meek, shy, and sensitive guy, wearing black clothing might give you a more masculine edge. However, if you are more macho, a little rough in your approach to women, then wearing a white shirt may soften your persona, making you more of a sweet tough guy. Every color has its own effect.

▶ *When in doubt, wear red.* —BILL BLASS

At the dawn of time, the earliest known Homo sapiens used red ocher to decorate and adorn themselves. Red is the color of passion and sensuality, and it has been shown to stimulate a faster heartbeat and faster breathing. It is often used in restaurants because it is considered to be an appetite stimulant. Because red is an emotionally intense color, it will make you stand out from the crowd and attract attention. Stop signals, brake lights, and fire hydrants are all painted red due to its visibility. No wonder red cars are the most popular targets for thieves and cops! Red has a life-affirming, positive association for most of us—after all, it is the color of our blood and our heart. Red is the color most commonly found in national flags, and in my native language, Russian, the word for *red* comes from the same root as the word for *beautiful*. Along with pink, red is also a color of love, so if you need to suggest that you are a romantic at heart, a little red or pink will sell that theme.

Pink has gotten a bad rap with a lot of guys, as it is considered to be a "girly" color. Sports teams sometimes paint the locker rooms used by opposing teams bright pink so their opponents will lose energy. Peach or even pink shades are not usually what macho men choose to wear, but they are missing a bet. Those colors not only convey the freshness of spring flowers but they also tell a woman that a man has an emotional, even feminine, side. Those hotties who are feminists and have had it up to here with all the macho types—and I freely admit to being one of them!—will welcome the approach of the sensitive man in peach.

▶ *When in doubt, wear blue.* —DR. Z

The color of the sky and the ocean, blue and all its shades and hues are popular with men and women. Studies have shown that women are attracted to men wearing blue. It is often seen as the opposite of red, and psychologically causes the opposite reaction. Peaceful and serene, light blue causes the body to produce calming chemicals. But beware—because blue is a cool color, deeper shades of blue could make you appear cold and serious. Blue also symbolizes loyalty and productivity—one study even showed that weight lifters were able to lift heavier weights in blue gyms. You will look more serious and conscientious in blue—that's why fashion consultants recommend wearing blue to job interviews. Similarly, navy denotes stability, respectability, and trust, and it should be a staple in a man's wardrobe, as women really look for these qualities. So, if in doubt, you can always wear a pair of cool blue jeans or a denim jacket.

Green, the most popular decorating color, symbolizes calm and composure, as it is the color of nature and forest greenery. It is considered to be easy on the eyes and can reportedly improve vision. TV stations and many hospitals use green in their rooms to soothe and relax broadcasters and patients. Light green is the color of spring and thus signifies youth, energy, and readiness to mate. Perhaps that is the reason why brides in the Middle Ages wore green to symbolize fertility! Dark green is more masculine and old-fashioned, and it implies wealth. It also tends to suggest wisdom, as nature has been around for a long time.

Brown is another earthy color, signifying peacefulness and solidity. It is reported to be more popular with men than women, but it happens to be one of my favorite colors for my fall and winter wardrobe. Light brown implies depth, maturity, and genuineness, but a lot of dark brown in your wardrobe can make you appear older, as wood, leather, soil, and decaying leaves all have shades of brown. Brown clothing looks great when combined with burnt orange and red during the fall and winter seasons, and with blue and turquoise during the summer. I am particularly fond of a guy who can pull off that Native American look of a brown or tan shirt, light blue jeans, and a wide leather belt with a turquoise buckle.

Yellow and orange are the colors of sun and fire. Yellow is an attention-getter, and it has been shown to speed up metabolism. It also increases alertness and concentration; that is why it is used for legal pads and Post-it notes. While light yellow clothes make one appear cheerful and optimistic, bright yellow is often perceived as overpowering and irritating. Studies have shown that people are more likely to lose their tempers, and crying babies are harder to soothe, in yellow rooms. Similarly to yellow, orange is best used sparingly in your wardrobe. A little bit shows you have spirit and spark; too much, and you are thought to be hot-tempered and dangerous.

Gray is a mixture of black and white, so it carries an air of mystery about it. A man in gray might be a tough guy or a nice guy, and so it keeps a woman guessing—which is often a good thing. You can also easily combine it with just about any other color.

Purple is the color of royalty, wealth, and sophistication, reminiscent of knights and duels. But because purple is rare in nature and associated with age and status, it can make you appear a bit artificial and pretentious. It should never be the predominant shade in your outfit.

Even if you have a great physique, unless you are at the gym or the beach, you are better off wearing a suit than a muscle shirt. Unlike men, who are attracted to women in provocative clothing, women judge men in tight-fitting or revealing clothes to be less attractive than fully clothed men because this relative undress signals that the man is interested only in short-term sex, according to evolutionary psychologists. The authors of the *Superman* comics had it backwards: in real life, Lois Lane would have been more attracted to nattily dressed Clark Kent than to the tights of the Man of Steel. Of course, the muscular physique and ability to leap tall buildings in a single bound might have overcome Lois's turnoff on the uniform; but unless you have Superman's powers, you will be better off in Armani suits than in tight-fitting garb or even Adidas sweats.

What a guy wears tells a woman a lot about his personality and fashion style, as well as his occupation, social status, maturity level, and grooming habits. If you are wearing grungy clothes and a baseball cap, you are unlikely to catch the eye of a hot girl. Discard anything your mother knitted or bought for you, as well as everything with stains, holes, or signs of wear and tear (unless they are cool jeans). Anything that is more than a few years old should be tossed as well. To keep looking stylish and in vogue, pick up men's magazines and check out the latest fashions. I also think that single-breasted jackets look much better than double-breasted ones (which only look good when they are buttoned). When it comes to jeans, ditch the low-rise ones. They give guys that pancake butt, and no woman wants to see a guy's crack when he bends over. Also, avoid wearing sports-team clothing—Derek Jeter doesn't wear his jerseys in public, and neither should you. And forget bargain shopping at K-Mart, JCPenney, or Gap. Average-looking clothes work for picking up average women but will probably not work for a majority of beauties. Finally, get an expensive watch. But when it comes to men wearing accessories, most hotties agree that less is more. Centerfolds Krista Ayne and Jamie Lynn both dislike it when a guy wears too much jewelry, and Playmate Charlotte Kemp equates gaudy jewelry with narcissism. To Pet Courtney Taylor, "if a man wore a necklace, or any jewelry besides a watch, that would be a big turn-off." You can opt for an interesting accessory such as an unusual belt buckle, ring, or bracelet, which will serve as *a conversation piece* for women you approach.

To dress well yet inexpensively, shop at designer outlet centers such as Neiman Marcus Last Call, Off Saks Fifth Avenue, Nordstrom's Last Call, Boss, etc. You cannot only find incredible deals on unique, designer items but you can also find some very hot women browsing for bargains (they are particularly popular with hot Eastern European chicks who are obsessed with fashion yet cannot afford exorbitant Madison Avenue prices). The other advantage to designer outlets is that you don't get annoying salespeople badgering you every three minutes. You can make a big mess trying on the clothing and not worry about the scornful eye of some stuck-up socialite. In fact, outlet shopping provides great opportunities for approaching women precisely because of the scarcity of sales clerks. If you see a hot chick, put on a jacket or another item of clothing and ask her what she thinks of it. Chances are, she will readily respond with her opinion. By doing this, you are demonstrating that you are a style-conscious guy and a guy who has a lot in common with a woman like her—and you're not afraid to solicit her opinion (a very desirable trait in a boyfriend). You can also use clothing items to draw attention to your particular body parts. If you have nice hands, ask her opinion while trying on gloves, or draw her attention to your large feet by asking what she thinks of the shoes you are trying on. Of course, you might not enjoy trying on clothes. If you really dislike clothes shopping, hire a personal shopper, or if that is out of your budget, ask a stylish female friend to accompany you on a shopping trip.

HIT	MISS
Straight-leg jeans	Pleated pants
Plain white T-shirt	Stained T-shirt with silly logo
Blue blazer	Sports-team clothing
Italian shoes	Sneakers
Expensive watch	Cheap bracelet
Cool beret	Baseball hat worn backwards
Tie that stands out	Bow tie
Socks that match pants	White socks with black pants
Motorcycle leather jacket	"Members-only" jacket
Color-coordinated outfit	Rainbow-colored outfit

PROBLEM	SOLUTION
Skinny neck	Thick tie
Thick neck	Open shirt
Big gut	Small belt buckle
Heavy	Dark shirt, dark suit, narrow tie
Short	Vertical pinstripes, tapered pant
Round face	Square glasses or shades
Square face	Round glasses or shades

Tip from the Scoring Experts *Beau Brummel was the eighteenth-century European fashion arbiter, a metrosexual man by today's standards. His allure came from his sense of style and meticulous attention to his appearance. He would spend several hours every morning scrubbing himself from head to toe in milk, water, and eau de cologne. He is credited with inventing the modern man's suit, worn with a tie; and he was rumored to take up to five hours to dress and polish his boots with champagne. Beau was the original "dandy," and his trendy threads brought many a hot woman to his bed.*

TIP #4: Dress fashionably by shopping at designer clothing outlets, and choose color schematics to complement your prototype. When you can't decide what to wear, wear blue, as it has been shown that women are attracted to men in blue. While shopping for clothes, look for opportunities to meet hot women by asking their opinion about the clothes you are trying on. ✦

Four

Self-Assurance:
Supersizing Your Confidence

I have no self-confidence. When girls tell me yes, I tell them to think it over.
　　　　　　　　　　　　　　　—RODNEY DANGERFIELD

Self-confidence or self-assurance is the most important personality trait any man can have for attracting a desirable woman. Indeed, a high level of self-confidence can overcome a lot of deficiencies in other areas; and without self-confidence, you may have no chance at all to score with a hot chick. This is because masculine self-confidence is subconsciously interpreted by women as a sign of virility, the ability to defend her and to sexually satisfy her, and often even status and resources. This interpretation is virtually universal; it is a powerful aphrodisiac; and it can lead a man with only average or below-average looks to bed the hottest women on the planet.

Here is one woman's story depicting how she was so impressed by a guy's display of self-confidence that she ended up sleeping with him that night (as reproduced from the book *The Evolution of Desire* written by renowned evolutionary psychologist David Buss):

I was sitting at a corner table talking to my girlfriend and sipping on a gin and tonic. Then Bob walked in. He walked into the bar like he owned the place, smiling broadly and very confident. He caught my eye and smiled. He sat down and started talking about how horses were his hobby. He casually mentioned that he owned a horse farm. When the last call for alcohol came, he was still talking about how expensive his horses were and said that we should go riding together. He said, "In fact, we could go riding right now." It was 2 a.m., and I left the bar and had sex with him. I never did find out whether he owned horses.

In fact, it was probably of little import whether this guy talked about horses, dogs, cars, sports, or anything else. After she noticed that he walked in "like he owned the place, smiling broadly and very confident," she had probably subconsciously made up her mind that he was a dominant alpha male and felt an instantaneous attraction to him.

I am the same way. When I was in law school, this cute blonde (admittedly not my first choice) guy in my class kept hitting on me, and I finally decided to go out with him. What a bummer! He turned out to be so indecisive, so full of excuses for every imagined imperfection, and so lacking in any basic self-confidence that I could hardly wait for the date to end. Needless to say, I did not go out with him again during my law school years. However, six years later, I ran into him at a club in New York City, and he had changed completely. Now working for a large law firm, he had his own place in the city and was brimming with self-confidence. Much to my surprise, I found myself attracted to him despite our past history, and we ended the night in his apartment. His looks hadn't changed in those six years, nor had his other personality traits, but that change from a seemingly insecure boy to a self-confident man made all the difference in how I related to him.

Indeed, virtually every Playmate and Pet I know rates self-confidence either first or among the top five qualities she looks for in a man. It is a universal lubricant for a woman's arousal. Not only does self-confidence translate into manliness in the female mind; you have to remember that many of these models have self-confidence issues of their own. The "take charge" kind of guy gets their joy juices flowing and fills their need to lean on a man to make decisions that they are afraid to make for themselves. Prince Charming, after all, is a prince—used to ordering people around and having servants fawning at him. The self-confident guy who snaps his fingers and gets waiters to hop to it, or who talks his way to the front of the line and the VIP table at nightclubs, is going to be a Prince Charming, indeed, for the typical centerfold hottie.

▶ *Macho doesn't prove mucho.* —ZSA ZSA GABOR

Many men attempt to feign self-confidence by putting on a false bravado, acting conceited, cocky, and arrogant, or bragging, boasting, or ostentatiously showing off. However, these tactics frequently backfire when they betray an "overcompensation" strategy. Women have an intuitive radar for guys' attempts to appear what they are not. As psychologist David Buss put it: "Women frequently distinguish false bravado from real self-confidence; the genuine article is more successful in attracting them." Believe me, I've been hit on by hundreds of these "cool and cocky" types, and I wouldn't give any of them the time of day. They might fool an average- or below-average-looking woman who doesn't ordinarily receive a lot of male attention, but they won't fool a woman who attracts a lot of men. So tell all those dating "gurus" or "coaches" who tell you to adopt a false cockiness to go back to their beer. You want to project real self-confidence!

▸ *Who has confidence in himself will gain the confidence of others.*
                                                    —*LEIB LAZAROW*

What is self-confidence? Mostly it is perceiving yourself as capable and worthy, of being able to achieve those things you set out to do. You can think of self-confidence as comprised of two factors: self-efficacy and self-acceptance. Self-efficacy is your belief in your ability to persist and accomplish your goals, whereas self-acceptance is your feeling of being valuable and capable and able to accept yourself the way you are. The combination of both comprises your self-esteem. Several studies have demonstrated that men who are high in self-esteem tend to approach physically attractive women and ask them for dates, regardless of their own physical attractiveness. Men who are low in self-esteem avoid approaching attractive women, believing that their chances are too slim.

Many men underestimate themselves—and overestimate what they believe is their "competition" for the girl of their dreams. When groups of men and women are shown the same pictures and asked to judge which male images are the hottest or most handsome, men often rate other men at least 25 percent higher in looks than women do. This is due to their fear that other men may be more handsome than they, and thus have a better chance with a good-looking woman. In fact, women are not all looking for male models or made-up movie stars. They often are more interested in a man who fits generally, but not necessarily perfectly, within their love maps, and who projects those personal qualities—primarily self-confidence—that tells them that this guy will be a good provider, lover, and potential father for her children. Thus, every guy who shies away from approaching a hottie because he doesn't think he is good-looking enough to interest her is wasting what may be a great opportunity.

▶ *Whether you think you can or think you can't, you're right.*

—*HENRY FORD*

Indeed, this is how false beliefs can create a self-fulfilling prophecy. For example, in the stock market, if it is widely believed that a crash is imminent, investors may lose confidence, sell most of their stock, and actually cause the crash. The same is true in the dating game: if you start with low self-esteem and assume you are going to fail even before you approach the woman you've been staring at all evening, if you bail completely, then you will never get to know if she could be attracted to you; and if you do make the approach, nervous and doubting yourself, you probably will lose her in the first ten minutes. Conversely, if you believe that you are capable of achieving what you set your mind to do—like scoring with hot women—you will approach her with a perceptible swagger, ready to sweep her off her feet; and if you truly believe yourself to be a capable, worthy individual, you will smile more, treat her with the right mixture of casual *insouciance* and interest, and give her the impression that you are a man who has "got his act together" and someone she wants to know. In that way your belief in yourself will actually create reality.

"Exhibit remarkable confidence and people will think your confidence comes from real knowledge. You will create a self-fulfilling prophecy: people's belief in you will translate into actions that help realize your visions. Any hint of success will make them see miracles, uncanny powers, the glow of charisma,"[16] says Robert Greene.

▶ *Keep on telling yourself that you have the confidence to score with hot women and your thoughts will become reality.*

> *One important key to success is self-confidence. An important key to self-confidence is preparation.* —ARTHUR ASHE

BUILDING YOUR SELF-CONFIDENCE

1. Make a list of your strong points. List all the positive things about yourself and the things that you believe are part of your character. Think of your innate talents, all the compliments you have received, or things that come easily to you. I am not talking here about particular accomplishments in particular occupations, schoolwork, or sports and the like. I am referring to personal attributes that define you as a person.

Here's a list of qualities from which you can choose to describe yourself: *Agreeable, Approachable, Artistic, Attentive, Calm, Capable, Caring, Cheerful, Clean, Compassionate, Concerned, Confident, Considerate, Cooperative, Decent, Dependable, Devoted, Enthusiastic, Flexible, Forgiving, Friendly, Generous, Gentle, Genuine, Good-natured, Grateful, Healthy, Helpful, Honest, Interesting, Kind, Level-headed, Loyal, Mature, Neat, Normal, Optimistic, Orderly, Passionate, Patient, Peaceful, Pleasant, Polite, Proud, Reasonable, Reverent, Sensitive, Sexy, Tender, Warm.*

When you have prepared your list, you have the qualities you want to believe define yourself. Keep the list close at hand. Frequently review this list to reinforce your belief in your strengths. Think about how a person with these qualities would act and behave, and emulate that behavior. Continually remind yourself of these good qualities, and try to project them in all your interpersonal activities, even on the Internet! Eventually, you will truly believe that you are in fact the person you want to be.

2. Learn unconditional self-acceptance. According to Rational Emotive Behavior Therapy (REBT), the key to feeling good about yourself is unconditional self-acceptance. Most of us judge ourselves, at least some of the time, on the opinions of others, expressed or not. To the extent we do so, we surrender our independence of thought and action, and become dependent on others to sustain our self-esteem. A better solution is to tell yourself that no opinion but your own is really important to you. Whether or not women see you as you are, as long as you believe you are a good person, you are such a person. Rational behavioral therapists call this "an elegant solution" when you can accept yourself regardless of the external factors in your life. For example, never think, *She's going to turn me down before I even ask for her number because I'm such a nerd.* Think instead, *If she turns me down, it may be bad luck—like I didn't happen to fit her love map—or her poor perception, but I am still a bright, intelligent guy with all the good qualities that beautiful women want.* Make a list of these so-called elegant solution statements about issues that you are now working on. When you catch yourself negating, doubting, or berating yourself, read these statements over and over.

3. Visualize yourself as confident even when you don't feel like it. Even if you feel particularly low on a particular day, it is often helpful to "fake it till you make it." Since our moods often follow our actions, try acting as if you are indeed fully confident. Acting that way might fool your brain into believing that you are actually feeling confident. For example, research has shown that when you force yourself to smile, you actually begin to feel happier (known as facial feedback hypothesis). This effect happens because there is a direct link between your face and your brain;[17] your facial muscles send a signal to your brain that you are smiling and your brain in turn interprets it as your positive mood. And research has found that when people are in a good mood, they are more creative and successful in problem solving.[18] To help your brain snap into confidence, visualize yourself as a confident, happy, relaxed alpha male, who captures the attention of women as he walks through the door.

4. Get rid of negative thoughts and replace them with positive ones. According to Cognitive Behavior Therapy (CBT), negative emotional states, like feeling unconfident, are accompanied by

internal thoughts that echo these emotions. Just the emotional fear
that you will strike out with a hot babe will start you thinking that
you are unworthy of her. However, that connection, while understandable, is not at all rational. Whether she likes you or not might
have nothing to do with you and everything to do with her, so
don't go around imagining that all of your fears about yourself are
imprinted on your T-shirt for every woman to see. Instead, identify
these negative thoughts or fears you have about yourself and your
abilities and replace them with positive ones. Look over the list
below, identify any of your own negative thoughts ("cognitions"),
then replace them with the corresponding positive affirmations.

NEGATIVE COGNITIONS	POSITIVE COGNITIONS
I don't deserve love	I can have love
I am worthless	I am worthy
I will fail	I can succeed
I am a disappointment	I am okay just the way I am
I cannot stand it	I can handle it
I should have done something	I did the best I could
I did something wrong	I learned from it

5. Stop "musturbation" and "shoulding" on yourself. REBT[19]
teaches that when people adopt absolutistic and rigid shoulds,
musts, and oughts, they very likely set irrational, impossible standards for themselves. Albert Ellis, the founder of Rational Emotive
Behavior Therapy, calls this practice of rigid demands "musturbation." In order to learn to accept yourself, you "must" stop demanding that you and others do things perfectly. So stop saying to
yourself *I must do this just like the book says* or *She ought to respond
to my opening this way* or *I should not have used that approach*. Those
absolutist assertions are only going to drain your self-confidence.
In fact, nobody's perfect. Accept that you will make mistakes from
time to time, and believe that in the end, you will achieve what

you set out to achieve. Indeed, tell yourself that the mark of a self-confident man is his ability to overcome his mistakes and press on toward his goals—and then do just that!

6. Surround yourself with positive, confident, and successful people. This will become a habit and one that will build confidence. You won't want to take your wimpy, lonely buddy with you when you are trying to pick up the hot honey you've set your sights on, so try to befriend the kind of guys who exhibit a high degree of self-confidence and who are positive about themselves. You can learn from them vicariously as you watch them approach women. However, watch out for the "fakes" who are mere braggarts. The "real" self-confident men don't have to impress others and don't brag about themselves or their conquests. In fact, they don't talk mainly about themselves as the ego-centered overcompensators do; they speak with authority and confidence on subjects of mutual interest. Confident men are men you quickly grow to respect—just like women do!

7. Replace global, internal attributions with situational, external ones. When we offer explanations about why things happened, we usually give one of two types of answers. One assigns causality to the external agent; i.e, "she is in a bad mood and that's why she ignored me." The other explanation is to blame yourself, internalizing the cause; i.e, "I said stupid things, that's why she rejected me." When you make yourself directly responsible for the event, you tend to get down on yourself. Moreover, if you tend to think that this is what will always happen, making it a global attribution as opposed to blaming the circumstances (situational attribution), you are likely to get outright depressed. In reality, all actions are usually caused by a combination of factors, many of which are out of our control. Accept that fact and never blame yourself for any failure you incur—external, situational, and temporary factors probably played a large role in it.

8. Change your locus of control and become an optimist. While it is important to realize that external factors play a large role in the outcome of events, it is equally important to believe that we still retain some control over our world and to remain optimistic. Those who believe that their efforts do make a difference in the outcome have internal locus of control and tend to be more confident in their success, work harder, and stay more motivated. Those who believe that their success is due largely to chance or luck tend to be less confident in their abilities to accomplish things.

Some people develop external locus of control and become pessimistic after a series of failures makes them lose faith in their ability to change their lives. If you tried to finish college several times and always flunked out, you might decide you will never succeed, stop trying, and stay in a job you detest. If you have been rejected by women over and over again, you might give up approaching them, thinking it is useless. This phenomenon, known as learned helplessness, was discovered by psychologist Martin Seligman. In a series of experiments with dogs, he noticed that some dogs that received a series of inescapable shocks gave up trying to escape when presented with the opportunity to do so, becoming helpless. However, not all dogs became helpless—about one-third did *not*, instead somehow managing to find a way out of the unpleasant situation in spite of their past experience with it. These optimistic dogs somehow managed to retain internal locus of control! If you want to become resistant to the shock of rejection, work on your optimism by telling yourself that your failures are not due to personal shortcomings, that they are limited to a small area of your life, and that you can change things around (your failures are not personal, pervasive, or permanent).

9. Avoid negative comparisons with other people. Each of us is unique, with our own sets of strengths and weaknesses—but all of us can be desirable to the opposite sex. Tom Cruise and Tommy Lee might seem to have an inside track at nailing all those hot Hollywood types, but many of their relationships have failed. Abraham Maslow, the main contributor to humanistic psychology, warned against comparing ourselves unfavorably with others and dwelling on our limitations.[20] You can follow Maslow's call to become a self-actualizing person by developing your own unique and creative talents. Review that list of good qualities that you have and pay no attention to whether other guys seem to be more successful. For all you know, they may be total losers in bed!

10. Adopt the "courage to be." Tell yourself that you don't really care what other people think of you, that as long as you are true to your own self-image (that list of good qualities, remember), you will be proud of yourself and your action, and that is all that counts. Don't be afraid to go against convention in order to accomplish your goals. You know what is right for yourself; what's more, you are not an "average" person or a blind follower of others. This "courage to be" will carry you through any situation, not just one involving women, but it has a profound effect on women who sense that you have it. It is the emotional equivalent of physical virility, and it is very sexy to even the most gorgeous, popular girls.

Maintaining your self-confidence and continuing to approach women, even when your advances are shot down, will set you apart from all your dejected competitors and will raise your odds of scoring with hot women. A truly self-confident man knows that he has the qualities that will prove enticing and endearing to attractive women, and that all he needs is a chance to show them. It may take some failures, even a lot of them, before he gets that chance, but I've never met a man with the real "courage to be" who has not ultimately succeeded.

Tip from the Scoring Experts *Grigori Rasputin, the scandalous nineteenth-century Russian monk and mystic, mesmerized women with his unwavering gaze and deep spell-binding voice. Women were drawn to this puzzling contradiction: his religious fervor juxtaposed with bla-*

tant lasciviousness. He would start preaching to a woman, then switch to whispering suggestive comments, and thus was perceived as saintly yet wicked, authentic yet mysterious, kind yet cunning, earning him the title "The Holy Devil." Despite having a shockingly ugly exterior, with a gangly body and stringy hair, Rasputin was self-confident and charismatic: an uninhibited dancer, a fiery prophet, and an unbridled seducer.

TIP #5: Develop self-confidence by:

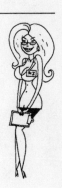

- Developing the "courage to be"

- Listing your positive traits

- Developing internal locus of control

- Learning unconditional self-acceptance

- Visualizing yourself as confident

- Replacing negative thoughts with positive ones

- Stopping "musturbation" and "shoulding"

- Emphasizing effort, not outcome

- Seeing uncertainty as a challenge ✦

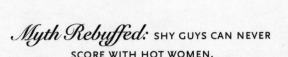

Myth Rebuffed: SHY GUYS CAN NEVER
SCORE WITH HOT WOMEN.

In fact, shyness is not an impediment to meeting hot women. "A man who is shy is not a turnoff, although it does make things a little awkward," states Pet Erica Ellyson. "My advice for a shy guy: Just ask her what her interests are, talk about things you like to do and just be yourself." Courtney Taylor echoes Erica's sentiments: "Shyness can be a turn-on, as long as it comes from introversion and not from being insecure. I love nervous chatter.

Like when a guy comes up and starts to talk about something totally mundane, like Seinfeld who just starts talking about the extra buttons on his shirt." According to Søren Kierkegaard, a glimpse of bashfulness can be very seductive because it disarms defenses that sexy women put up against aggressive men, lulling these women into a state of trust and comfort.

Five

Fear of Rejection:
Reaching Rejection Immunity State

REACHING REJECTION IMMUNITY STATE (OR RIS)

Everyone risks being laughed at when he approaches a woman.
That is always at stake. Take a chance . . . and if worse comes
to worse, let yourself be laughed at.

—HERMANN HESSE, *Steppenwolf*

Some guys who are very confident in other aspect of their lives get so nervous when they attempt to meet women that they end up blowing it. A little anxiety in approaching people we do not know is normal and natural; after all, we never know how the person we approach is going to react. For men, feeling anxious about approaching a woman may have evolutionary underpinnings, as hitting on women was a dangerous practice in ancestral times, when most women were the property of a tribal leader. Thus, your predecessors risked being physically assaulted if they approached a woman who belonged to another male. Although this risk is virtually nonexistent today, your brain has been programmed by years of evolution for a fight-or-flight reaction when approaching women. In reality, the worst outcome of your approach to a beautiful woman is her polite refusal to chat with you. We live in a civil society, and very few women are rude to men who approach them. In fact, unless you are uncouth, sexually harassing, or menacing to them, most hot women are flattered by men approaching them, because it is an affirmation of their attractiveness, which they constantly seek. So whenever you feel nervous approaching a woman, remind yourself that chances of her being rude to you are very low.

▸ *Men are evolutionarily programmed to be fearful to approach women.*

Another reason men experience such intense anxiety is their engagement in what psychologists call dysfunctional or negative cognitions. Examples of these negative thoughts are *catastrophizing* (imagining the worst possible outcome), *awfullizing* (telling themselves how awful it is to be rejected by a woman), and *exaggerating* (imagining your conversational skills to be far worse than they are).

To counteract your tendency to exaggerate and catastrophize, look at the Catastrophe Scale below. If real catastrophes, such as nuclear war or a meteorite striking the earth, are 100, and getting in a car accident is 50, then where does being rejected by a woman lie? Somewhere close to a zero! This should help put your fear of approaching women in perspective!

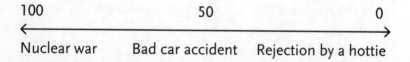

100	50	0
Nuclear war	Bad car accident	Rejection by a hottie

If even thinking of approaching a hot woman makes you break out in a cold sweat, you need to practice some cognitive restructuring followed by lots of practice. Learn to identify these automatic negative thoughts that enter your mind when you see a hot woman. Then actively "talk back," or rebut them, with positive, logical statements. Think of yourself as a control tower operator who talks through the landing process for an airplane pilot, or a coach who helps an athlete through a new experience.

When you rebut your dysfunctional thoughts, remember that your rebuttals must be strong and specific. When you feel yourself getting anxious and doubts begin to enter your mind, choose a forceful, dominant voice and say to yourself "STOP IT! You are OK, you can do it. Just because you didn't know what to say last time doesn't mean you will falter now!" This technique is also known as Thought Stopping. You can also include a physical act like snapping your fingers, whistling to yourself, or tweaking a rubber band placed around your wrist to interrupt a negative train of thought.

Practice challenging your fears using this exercise:

What's the Evidence Exercise

My anxiety is:
Acting stupid when approaching a woman.

What evidence supports this idea?
I get nervous and act stupid.

What evidence goes against the idea?
It doesn't mean I look stupid when I act nervous.

Show me the logic:
Being nervous makes me look stupid.

Is there a cause-and-effect connection?
Not really.

Am I accurate or exaggerating?
Yeah, I am exaggerating.

Am I looking at it in all-or-nothing terms?
Yes.

Am I confusing "possible" with "probable"?
Yes. It's possible I look stupid.

Am I judging on my feeling or on facts?
On my feelings.

Another way to combat fear of rejection is by brainstorming other interpretations of the situation. If you are really down on yourself because some hottie declined your invitation to lunch, try to take her point of view. One reason why she declined your offer could be that you are not her type. But what are alternative theories? She might have a boyfriend, or she might be going through a man-hating phase, or you might remind her of her estranged father, or she might be feeling unattractive, or just having a bad day. Or maybe she is a gold digger or a call girl and is only interested in sex for money. Or maybe she is a lesbian, or a transvestite. There are many possible explanations for why she turned you down.

You can also combat your negative cognitions by using a reframing technique. Think of your life as a painting that is hanging on the wall. It is a painting of a horse standing by a rose fence with mountains and green pastures in the background. Where you place your frame in this panorama will determine what picture you see. You can choose to see the whole picture and focus on the pastures that lie ahead, or you can focus on the front of the horse next to the roses, or on the horse's behind. The next time you see the situation as bleak (i.e., "this woman rejected me—my life sucks"), remind yourself to take a broader picture and get away from the horse's behind.

▶ *What the mind perceives, the mind believes, so visualize yourself being confident with women.*

By gaining control of your imagery, you can gain control over your fear of rejection. Research has shown that our brain does not differentiate between fantasized images and images that come from reality. In fact, "what the mind perceives, the mind believes." One version of the visualization technique is called Time Projection. It is especially useful when you get anxious anticipating an event, such as approaching a hot coworker to ask her out. To manage your anxiety, visualize yourself successfully approaching her. Watch your actions, speech, and behavior, and see her responding to you. Because you cannot predict what her response will be, the key is to visualize yourself successfully handling both acceptance and rejection. The time projection technique is often used by athletes to improve their performance.

Another visualization technique is called TV-set Technique. Think of your mind images as the ones you see on a TV set. If you don't like what you see (i.e., you as a nervous wreck), you can always change the channel or tune it out. Now take it a step further and imagine yourself to be a producer of the TV soap opera of your life. You write the script and audition the actors. If you don't like the way a hottie is acting in your play, you can simply fire her and move on to another one—until you cast the right one for the role.

You can also use humor to help you overcome your anxiety. Research has shown that laughter helps release anxiety-controlling hormones in your system. Whenever you begin to take the situation too seriously, just step back and find something funny about it. Try to look at the whole thing from a TV sitcom writer's point of view and have a good laugh.

Another reason a lot of guys panic and stop short of approaching a woman is that they think that women can tell just how nervous they are. Remember, a woman does not know about the self-doubts racing in your head, she has no idea that you have butterflies in your stomach, and your outward signs of nervousness are not as visible as you think they are. Most of us exaggerate how bad our anxiety makes us look. Many times when I appeared on national TV I was a total nervous wreck. I felt that I was blushing, that my voice was trembling, and that I did not sound as clever as I wanted to, due to my anxiety. But my friends and fans who watched me on TV thought I did just great—and many times, once I watched the show later, I would be surprised to find just how little my anxiety showed! If anything, it made me look more real and authentic, and more likeable.

In fact, a little anxiety has been shown to improve people's performance and students' scores on tests. It is when your perception of the threat level is so exaggerated that it prevents you from doing what you want to do that anxiety becomes dysfunctional. You may never get rid of your approach anxiety completely, but you can get to the point where you can perform well despite it. Ask yourself, What is the worst that could happen if I get rejected. Then remind yourself that the only thing to fear is fear itself. Here's another useful exercise to help you get over catastrophizing, exaggerating, and awfullizing:

The So-What Exercise

I fear that this will happen:
She will laugh in my face.

So what if it happens?
I will be embarrassed.

Then what can I do?
Go back to my friends.

And then what will happen?
They will make fun of me.

So what if it happens?
I will feel like crap about myself.

Then what can I do?
Get over it.

What is the worst thing that will happen?
I will get rejected and made fun of.

Do this exercise often, substituting your own worries and anxieties, and you will see that rejection is not a big deal. It won't kill you, and you will get over it soon enough.

▸ *Laugh at yourself, but don't ever aim your doubt at yourself. Be bold. When you embark for strange places, don't leave any of yourself safely on shore. Have the nerve to go into unexplored territory.*

—ALAN ALDA

Getting control over your negative cognitions is just the first step in reaching the Rejection Immunity State. The next step is to go out and overcome your rejection anxiety through practice. There is no substitute for practice, whether in scoring with women or scoring on the gridiron. The more you try, the more likely it is you will succeed. However, one of the hardest things for most guys is to maintain their self-confidence despite repeated rejection by women. According to one study, men rebuffed by women in their first few attempts produced successively less confident approaches. The psychological discomfort of rejection caused the men to experience resentment and hostility and to lower their sights to women who have lower appeal.[21]

Albert Ellis, the founder of Rational Emotive Behavior Therapy, or REBT, claims to have overcome his own dating anxiety by approaching hundreds of women on the street. Similarly, to help his clients get over their anxiety, he told them to approach strangers on the street and ask them, "I just got out of the mental hospital, what time is it?" or do even more embarrassing things such as pretend to walk a banana on a string in the park, then sit down on a bench next to an attractive woman and pretend to feed a banana to your banana on a string. The point of these exercises is to see that embarrassment is not nearly as scary or catastrophic as we believe it to be. Most of Ellis's patients found that the more they practiced this exercise, the less anxious and the more amused they became. As a matter of fact, they noticed that the bystanders became more uncomfortable than the people performing bizarre behaviors!

Of course, you don't have to walk your banana on a string to learn to meet women (although it would make a great conversation piece!). If you want to desensitize yourself to rejection in a slow and systematic way, start practicing under less stressful conditions. Begin by talking to all sorts of strangers: UPS delivery guys, waiters, guys who park next to you, old ladies walking their dogs, cashiers at a grocery stores, etc, etc. Just smile and make a comment—about anything. Most of the time strangers will smile and say something back. Once you are comfortable talking to guys and old ladies, begin approaching average or below-average women. Try sampling different ethnic and age categories to see how different women react; try picking up the Asian manicurist at the nail salon, or approaching women at a Hispanic nightclub. Approaching foreign women will give you an idea of how women from different cultures react to you. You might find that Asian women find you too direct, while Eastern European women love your style. The more different women you meet, the more you will be able to anticipate different types of reactions.

See if you can have a nice conversation with a female neighbor or the girl behind the counter at Starbucks. She doesn't have to be a beauty, and you don't have to pick her up or take her out—just see if you can capture her interest for five minutes. Then try it with another girl, and another, until you feel that you can talk to any woman. Then you can ask out that Starbucks girl and see how it goes. Every time you do succeed, the next time is easier; and you can use the memory of each success to plan your next move. When you feel like you have it down, you can take on the supermodel you've had your eyes (and mind) on.

▸ *You can't score if you keep your bat on your shoulder.*

—CASEY STENGEL

If your anxiety does not subside after practicing all of the above, you might want to consult your doctor for a possible antianxiety medicine. Use it at the beginning to give yourself courage to approach women, then, as your confidence grows, just keep it in your pocket as a safety token.

DEMYSTIFY THE POWER OF HER SEX APPEAL

▸ *Beauty is in the eye of the beholder.*

Finally, some guys do just fine approaching average and even cute women but become totally tongue-tied when facing that stunning, supersexy hottie. Indeed, research has shown that male brains are strongly influenced by hot women. In one study, men were far more likely to buy things they did not need from sexy women than from average-looking ones. And the men with the highest testosterone level were most susceptible to such clouded judgment. It is as if hotties mesmerize men, obliterating all rational thought and willpower!

To become facile at picking up hot women, you need to get over the power that their looks have over you. You need to demystify beauty in your eyes. One of the most important principles in approaching and dating beautiful women is this: don't be intimidated by their beauty. Act totally unaffected by their sex appeal. This is the ironic truth—sexy women are attracted to men who are not affected by their sex appeal. A hot woman who feels that a guy is not smitten by her sex appeal is like a frustrated fairy who discovers that her magic wand does not work on him—she will be drawn to capture his heart even if just to prove to herself that her magic still works. Whenever a hot woman feels that her looks are turning you into Jell-O, you will lose that mystique and will no longer be a challenge to her. You will be like all the other horny guys that follow her like hungry puppies. On the contrary, the more you come across as a connoisseur of beauty, the more attracted she will be to you. A beauty connoisseur is someone who has scored with other hot women and who can truly appreciate beauty without being blinded by it. Your attitude should project *I have been around beautiful women and I prefer beauties with substance. No matter how hot you are, I won't be with you unless you demonstrate to me your substantive value.* Coming from this position, you can let her validate herself to you as having more than sex appeal. Even if she seems breathtakingly beautiful to you, do not show how smitten you are. If you do, you will lose your control over the situation, giving her too much power at the start. Instead of coming across as a worldly guy who has been around hot women and who knows how to satisfy them in bed, you will come across as a wide-eyed novice.

At the beginning, this will be very difficult for you, because beauty has a subconscious influence on our behavior. Some women are so hot that they take your breath away. Your mind unconsciously reads beauty as truth and goodness—you know the adage "Beauty is truth, truth is beauty." For centuries, female youth and health signified fertility and fecundity to our ancestral males, thus programming the male mind to find female characteristics that indicate youth and health to be beautiful. Evolution has taught men to subconsciously respond to female beauty with excitement and arousal. Due to this effect, you need to consciously resist this awe-inspiring influence of beauty on your judgment.

If you feel yourself being impressed by her beauty or affected by her sex appeal, take a minute to "deconstruct" her good looks. Imagine her without makeup, with oily hair, sitting on the toilet, passing gas, and picking her nose—trust me, even the hottest women do it! Then think of all the ways in which she tried to enhance her looks. If her hair is blond, chances are very high that she highlights it, and if it is long, she might have extensions.

She probably puts on foundation to cover her blemishes and skin imperfections and wears mascara or even fake lashes to make her eyes stand out. Imagine her in twenty, thirty, forty years, as her beauty fades and she no longer has the same effect on you. What else will she have to offer you? Think of how hot Britney Spears looked—until she became bald.

Things to Tell Yourself to Resist the Effect of Beauty on Your Judgment

+ Beauty is in the eye of the beholder

+ Beauty is temporary and fleeting

+ Beauty doesn't equal goodness

+ Beauty is empty without substance

+ Beauty can be artificially created

+ Beauty is not enough for me

Once you demystify the power of beauty, you will be able to act with a lot more ease around hot women.

If you find yourself becoming nervous when facing an attractive woman, use this visualization technique. Imagine that instead of talking to this hottie, you are talking to your grandmotherly neighbor. Envision her disheveled gray hair, her dirty apron, as she is offering you her slightly burnt baked cookies. Chances are you will feel far less nervous. And if she ends up rejecting you, remind yourself that you are a fully qualified candidate, and that if she didn't like you, you are probably not her ideal prototype.

TIP #6: To get over your anxiety and develop the Rejection Immunity State (RIS):

• Stop "catastrophizing" and "awfullizing"

• Challenge your anxiety by questioning your logic

• Ask yourself, "What's the worst that could happen if I get rejected? So what?"

• Desensitize yourself against rejection by meeting

lots of different women

• Visualize talking to your grandmother instead

• Find something humorous about anxiety-provoking situations

• Demystify beauty by imagining what a hottie will look like in fifty years

• Practice, practice, practice! ✦

Six

Coolness and Kindness: Being Strong but Sensitive

Looks don't concern me, Maestro. Only talent interests a woman of taste. —KATERINA CAVALIERI in *Amadeus*

In addition to self-confidence, there are other internal qualities that appeal to women. All are just as important as your external attributes. Studies have shown that women express a greater preference than men do for a wide array of socially desirable personality traits.[22] While men seem to have two lists of things that they desire in a woman—one is focused on looks for a one-night stand, the other is focused on looks and personality for a long-term relationship—women have just one list. They want a man to be confident, caring, intelligent, and understanding, even for just a one-night stand.

This preference for a "strong but sensitive" guy may have evolutionary roots that are deeply embedded in the female psyche. Women were much more likely to be targets of violence back in the cavemen times, and they looked for strong and kind men who could offer them, and their progeny, support and protection. Studies have shown that women accord more weight than men do to nonphysical characteristics of prospective partners, such as ambitiousness, character, and intelligence—traits that would maximize survival of potential progeny.[23]

What that means for you is that you are unlikely to get that hottie to fall for you if you act like a cruel, insensitive, unstable jerk, no matter how rich and handsome you are. But don't be frightened—you don't have to possess all of the positive qualities women find desirable, although the more of them you possess the higher rating you will receive by desirable women. And being able to cultivate and display these qualities is totally under your control.[24]

HUMOR/WIT—YOUR FUNNY BONE

Almost universally, women are attracted to guys who are funny, witty, and have a good sense of humor. In fact, almost every model I know or have interviewed has listed "sense of humor" as one of the top qualities she seeks in her man. Penthouse Pet Courtney Taylor is so into having her funny bone tickled that she requires the men she dates to be aficionados of Woody Allen movies, as she gets off on his quirky brand of humor. In fact, she admitted to me that she would love to hook up with Woody himself, so infatuated is she with his wit. (See, what did I tell you: having the "right stuff" as far as hot women are concerned can overcome almost any deficiency in the looks department.) This preference is not just confined to models and centerfolds. A recent psychological study in which college women were presented with photos of men with either witty autobiographies or serious ones rated the "funny" men as more romantically desirable than plain talkers. To put it simply: if you can make her laugh, you have already garnered some major points on her dating scorecard.[25]

But what does having a sense of humor really mean? Obviously, not everyone can crack jokes the way Chris Rock or David Letterman can, and very few guys are endowed with Jim Carrey's talent for making goofy faces. But anybody can learn a few good jokes or recall funny situations or events that happened to them in their past. Being able to get her laughing over the crazy antics of your nutty brother or goofball friends has two salutary effects: it boosts her endorphin levels and it gets her talking about family and friends too. Think of it this way: you can tell her what you are like, what you are looking for in a woman, or what interests you have, etc., in a serious voice, full of drama and portentousness; and she might think you are a real loser. But give her the same information packaged in laughter, and she will think you're a "real man."

The essence of the humor you should strive for is that which makes her feel comfortable and relaxed with you. Stay away from racist, ethnic, sexist, political, religious, and sexually explicit jokes until you get to know her well enough to avoid pushing any sensitive buttons she might have. For example, Polish people are close to my native Ukrainians, so I don't like "dumb Polack" jokes. On the other hand, I don't mind "dumb blonde" jokes, because let's face it, a lot of these platinum-haired, big-chested bunnies are pretty dumb. But you need to know me a little to be able to make that distinction. So, if you've got an arsenal of "dumb blonde" jokes, ask your girl her opinion of Anna Nicole Smith. If she starts off her response with "that gold-digging bimbo . . ." you know you can unload your jokes on her.

▸ *Humor is a universal turn-on for women.*

I believe self-deprecating jokes are always safer than those deprecating others, which can easily backfire if you don't know the woman you are talking to. You can also tease or playfully mock her, as long as you don't cross over into the boundary of put-downs, sarcasm, or cynicism. Although there is a fine line between humor and sarcasm, sarcasm has been described as "anger with a smile," and anger is not what you want to project. Few women appreci-

ate sarcastic remarks, especially if they have to do with her appearance, and very especially if they are about an artificial, surgically
enhanced or fake aspect of her appearance. So, if you approach a
woman who seems somewhat overdressed and say, "That's a great
dress you're wearing; are you going to a wedding today?" you can
get away with it; but "That's a great dress—it really makes your
boobs look like big melons" is likely to gain you a big "F" on your
report card.

Ways of Displaying Humor

HIT	MISS
Original/subtle	Canned/obvious
Self-deprecating	Putting down others
Verbal jokes	Practical jokes
Teasing jokes	Mocking, mean ones
Ironic jokes	Sarcastic or cynical ones

MAGNANIMITY/KINDNESS—YOUR BIG HEART

If the "big" word *magnanimity* scares you, simply think of it as the
opposite of being petty. A dictionary definition of *magnanimity* is
"extremely liberal generosity of spirit" or "generosity in overlooking
injury or insult." Its synonyms are *bigheartedness, freehandedness,
generosity, liberality, openhandedness,* and *unselfishness.* Generosity
is the main idea behind this concept, and yes, that means not
being stingy with your money, although it goes far beyond material possessions. One study found that men who bought more
expensive drinks for the women they tried to pick up in bars were
more successful than those who bought cheaper drinks (mixed
drinks, being more expensive, worked better than beer or wine).
Picking up the tab, leaving large tips, paying for her parking and

(later) surprising her with nice gifts and getaways is included in this concept.

I was once out on a date with a man I was intensely, madly attracted to. He was a handsome and wealthy surgeon who perfectly fit my "love map." We were strolling on the streets of Manhattan, and it began to drizzle. I was wearing an expensive dress and matching high heels, which had begun to hurt my feet. There were no available cabs, but a limo pulled up offering his services. My date inquired as to how much the limo ride was and, upon finding out it was $25, dismissed the limo—making me walk in the rain, in painfully high heels. Needless to say, his cheapness immediately put a damper on the fire of my desire. Here was a doctor who made $25,000 an hour doing surgery, and he couldn't spend $25 on a ride?

Cheapness is a universal turn-off. In his book *The Art of Seduction*, Robert Greene lists lack of generosity as one of the most repelling qualities because "being unable to give by spending money usually means being unable to give in general. . . . Try giving more freely of both your money and yourself and you will see the seductive potential in selective generosity."[26]

Kindness is a quality related to magnanimity, and some would even classify it as part and parcel of magnanimity. In one international study, women of all thirty-seven cultures studied ranked kindness as one of the three most important qualities in a mate, out of a possible thirteen qualities.[27] And on the questionnaire I gave to my centerfold friends, "kindness" was rated almost as high as "confidence," which was rated the most highly desirable quality in a man.[28]

How do you display your kindness? By being thoughtful and considerate of the needs of others. In one singles bar study by the prominent evolutionary psychologist David Buss, women stated that the most effective tactics a man can use to attract them are: displaying good manners; offering help; and acting sympathetic and caring. Buss went on to conclude that "mimicking what

women want in a husband by showing kindness and sincere interest . . . is also an effective technique for luring women into brief
sexual liaisons."

You can also show your kind side through charitable deeds. I
was once walking on the streets of Manhattan when I saw a young
man who had bent down to collect the scattered objects of a sleeping homeless man. The young man caught my attention, and we
ended up striking a conversation. His willingness to stop and help
the homeless man really touched me and made me perceive him
as a good person worth knowing. You can work on developing your
charitable side by helping out at the Humane Society or homeless
shelters or volunteering at a children's hospital. Doing charity
work in your spare time will not only provide you with an opportunity to meet women but will also give you plenty of conversational
material with women.

▶ *Women love kind, nurturing men, so show off your magnanimity of
spirit by getting involved in charities.*

Displaying concern and nurturance toward the young is an
extremely effective male tactic for attracting women. In one study,
women were shown slides of the same man in three different
conditions—standing alone, interacting positively with a baby,
and ignoring a baby in distress. Women were most attracted to
the man when he was acting kindly toward the baby.[29] So if you
have an opportunity to show off your nurturance toward kids or
animals in front of attractive women, by all means do so. I knew a
man who met a number of attractive single mothers by taking his
little nephew to a kid's gym. The man was funny and entertaining and knew how to mimic voices of Disney characters; naturally,
kids would flock to him, and so did their cute single mothers. Little did these MILFs (an acronym for "mothers I'd like to fuck")
know that he had no intention of settling down and having kids of
his own!

Owning pets like cats and dogs is also a big plus. Women, by and large, are animal lovers; and good-looking women are even more so. Pets for Pets is the biggest charity that Penthouse Pets get involved in; many models have their own animal charities too. A cute cat or dog is a great prop to use in meeting women, as it provides a good topic for conversation, and it marks you as a kind, caring type of guy. Subconsciously, of course, the woman will be judging your fitness for fatherhood on how you care for your pet; so it gives you a chance to show your kindness factor without having to change a diaper.

EQUANIMITY/STABILITY—YOUR COOLNESS FACTOR

Equanimity is another fancy word, which really means "coolness." Its synonyms are *evenness of mind, calmness,* and *composure.* This means keeping your cool when a rival insults you or spills a drink on you, and not flying off the handle when a distracted driver cuts you off. This also encompasses dependability, mental stability, and maturity. In an international study of female preferences, among the eighteen characteristics rated, the second and third most highly valued male personality traits were a dependable character and emotional stability or maturity. Women are evolutionarily programmed to select males for these qualities, the authors of the study concluded, because choosing undependable, emotionally unstable men would have threatened the survival of the ancestral woman. In our times, equanimity and dependability continue to have an appeal to women. A dependable, stable, mature guy will call when he promised to and will not fly off the handle in a jealous rage. He will not fall apart when a problem arises or curl into a fetal position or seek the proverbial nipple to turn to.

I was out on a date with a guy, having drinks in a local bar, when a fight broke out. Not only were fists flying but the fighters had also drawn knives. My date, however, was a picture of coolness through the whole thing, protecting me from any potential danger, as well as talking the fighters out of any bloodshed. I can't tell you how impressed I was with his equanimity, and I made sure *he* knew how impressed I was that very night!

The bottom line: women want to deal with an adult, not a whiney infant. Lack of equanimity or mental stability also suggests a bad temper—or a potential stalker. Another reason why women appreciate dependability and stability in a guy is that these are good signs of his ability to commit—and women really hate commitment phobia in a man!

▸ *Show her what a stable, reliable, mature guy you are and her attraction to you will grow exponentially.*

You can acquire the kind of equanimity women want by acquiring self-confidence in your ability to handle most situations. You don't have to be a James Bond, a study in coolness even when being attacked by a horde of megalomaniacal killers; but you should be able to remain calm in the midst of a traffic jam, even though it's going to make you late for the show, or have the presence of mind to call when you learn that you will be late picking her up. Many beautiful women end up marrying or bedding older men, and it's not just for their money. Their ability to remain calm, collected, deliberate, and purposeful even in times of stress or crisis is very attractive to women!

Learning to control your temper is another important step in attracting hot women. With their obsession with beauty and their feelings of entitlement, such women may be especially sensitive to angry words or intemperate actions. What may be just an ordinary "disagreement" in a normal relationship can be blown up into a major scene by the ego sensitivity in the head of a supermodel. Therefore, maintaining your cool in the midst of trouble or strife is critical to maintaining a relationship with a hot honey;

and showing you have this ability is a good way to win a favorable impression from her. So, every chance you get, you should try to be Mr. Cool.

Ways of Displaying Stability

HIT	MISS
Calm reaction to an aggressive driver	Calm reaction to a nasty drunk
Ignoring some guy flirting with her	Ignoring her flirting with some guy
Calling when promised	Being obsessively punctual

AMBITION/INDUSTRIOUSNESS— YOUR SKY-HIGH DREAMS

As I have mentioned before, you don't have to be rich or have a great job to date hot women. However, most desirable women want a guy who enjoys working, is motivated to advance in life, and who has some goals and ambitions. Studies indicate that women worldwide are attracted to men who enjoy their work, show career orientation, demonstrate industriousness, and display ambition. In one study, women rated men who lack ambition as extremely undesirable—whether for a long-term relationship or even a short-term fling! It's the old "can he take care of me" thing, inbred in women since the days of primitive tribal hunting societies. So even if you don't have a good job, or are unemployed at the present time, you'll want to tell her about your future career ambitions and how much you look forward to working toward them.

▶ *Talking about your ambitions is a great way to capture a woman's attention.*

Discussing your life ambitions is always a great idea, as women love charismatic men. If your ambitions also encompass kindness, so much the better, as you can tally twice on her love interest board. If you aspire to be a doctor, volunteer fireman, paramedic, veterinarian, or any health care professional, play it for all it is worth. You don't have to have a great job to impress a woman, but you should sound enthusiastic about your job. Think of all the positive aspects of your occupation, and be prepared to discuss them with zeal.

You can also demonstrate your masculinity and self-confidence through the loftiness of your ambitions. Tell her how you plan to earn a black belt in karate, run for office, climb Mount Everest, save an endangered species, or discover the lost city of Atlantis! She might not believe that you will succeed at such things, but she will have a good impression of you anyway. If they have some secondary appeal, even small ambitions can be positive such as planting a tree (this shows you respect the environment and nature, which women find to be nurturing) or writing a book on a subject she is interested in or even in being a good father some day (we've seen what an important subconscious connection this one is).

Never let her think you are a couch potato or aspire to win the lottery and spend your time playing video games. Being seen as a lazy bum is the kiss of death for dating a hot model or any beautiful woman. Their "narcissistic entitlement" streak and their ability to pick and choose widely will automatically lead them to believe that they are entitled to more in a man. Plus, they get plenty of propositions from men seeking to use them. And their high-maintenance shopping habits mean that they will expect a man who is able to afford them. So, if you want to score with a centerfold, aim high with your ambitions and let her know that you dream of success in work as much as in play.

Ways of Displaying Ambition

HIT	MISS
Telling her your job goals	Talking only about your job
Telling her you work a lot	Telling her that work is your life
Sharing your job enthusiasm	Complaining about your job

CHIVALRY/COURTESY—YOUR KNIGHTLY NATURE

Chivalry is another one of those familiar words that most people have difficulty defining. Its meaning stems from medieval times and encompasses the noble qualities a knight was supposed to have, such as courage, justice, loyalty, humility, gallantry, courtesy, and a readiness to help the weak. Those who demonstrate these qualities are referred to as chivalrous. In modern times, chivalry is most frequently interpreted as attentiveness and courteousness with respect to women. This also encompasses good manners—opening and holding a door for her, pulling out her chair, waiting to start your meal until hers is served—all those masculine manners that were known to your fathers and grandfathers.

Many men wrongly believe that chivalry is not appreciated in the post-feminist era. However, most women of today yearn for displays of courteousness and attentiveness, no matter how financially independent or liberated they are. I am one of the most ardent feminists you are ever likely to meet; yet it turns me off when a man fails to hold a door for me or starts chomping away on his steak without waiting for me to be served. I have heard more complaints from my fellow models about simple obnoxiousness than about almost anything else. Lack of manners is very close to lack of common courtesy, and women do not appreciate discourteousness in a man. Indeed, some centerfolds I know have said they judge a man by how he treats his mother—which foretells the kind of courtesy and chivalry they might expect as his girlfriend.

▶ *The world's male chivalry has perished out, but women are knights-errant to the last; and, if Cervantes had been greater still, he had made his Don a Donna.*   —*ELIZABETH BARRETT BROWNING*

You have to remember that a majority of little girls still grow up reading the princess stories, hoping that one day they'll encounter their "knight in shining armor." Along with their love maps of what their prince looks like, these little girls grow up hoping to meet their chivalrous knight. So, chivalry is not dead in the twenty-first century; you can score with courtesy as well as muscles and good looks.

However, one caveat needs to be mentioned here. The line between true chivalry and fawning solicitousness is a somewhat narrow one. Being overly ingratiating, bringing her things every minute, trying too hard to impress her—these can be negative characteristics, destroying the impression of chivalry you are trying to create. I have had several fans who brought me flowers wherever I made public appearances, who always wanted to bring me drinks or food while I signed autographs, and who generally made a nuisance of themselves. These guys would not have had a chance with me; fortunately, they lacked the self-confidence to even ask. So don't go too far in this regard. Also, true chivalry extends to all women, from waitresses in restaurants to the friends of the woman you are interested in. If you want to impress her with your chivalry, you have to show it to all, not just to her.

INDEPENDENCE/AUTONOMY—
YOUR DISCARDED APRON STRINGS

There is no doubt that women are attracted to men who have a great sense of personal independence. An independent male does not seek the approval of others, and he is not affected by their opinions. He can be a maverick, a nonconformist, a radical, yet he is never a yes-man. He does not seek to ingratiate himself with a beautiful woman and is not afraid to disagree with her on occasion. An independent male is appealing to a woman because he is unlikely to be clingy, overly possessive, or jealous. He is unlikely to monopolize her time, or get upset over her need to spend time with her girlfriends and family. Psychologists call this type of personal independence a "strongly differentiated sense of self."

▶ *Show her that you are a self-reliant guy who can take care of himself—and her.*

On the other hand, one of the biggest turnoffs for women are men who are overly dependent on their parents or other family members. This does not mean it is bad to be close and affectionate to your family, but if you are dependent on their opinion in most, if not all, of your decisions, or if you are constantly seeking their approval, you will be perceived as a weak, ineffectual, and wimpy kind of guy by most women. You can secretly cherish your emotional umbilical cord with your mother, but under no circumstances reveal it to your hot date. I was with a guy once who pulled out his cell phone, dialed his mother, and then asked me to say hello to her—on the first date! I almost dumped him then and there. There will be a time to introduce your hot girlfriend to your family, but it comes long after the introduction, the first couple of dates, and the first couple of months of sex.

INTELLIGENCE/ERUDITION—YOUR BRAINIER SIDE

Although intelligence is harder to define than some of the other characteristics, women clearly prefer smarter guys. An international study on mate preferences revealed that women rate education and intelligence fifth out of eighteen desirable characteristics. And analysis of Playmate data sheets reveals that intelligence is listed as one of the most frequent turn-ons.[30]

Erudition is a subtype of intelligence—it is informational knowledge. Guys who know a lot about various topics and are able to comment easily on them make entertaining, exciting conversationalists. And exciting women like men who keep them excited. I am always impressed with men with large vocabularies and volumes of interesting information on all kinds of topics. I even find erudite men to be sexy, even if they don't always fit my love map profile. I even hooked up with one of my law school professors, who was not my type physically but who excited my imagination with his breadth of knowledge and his confident, dramatic delivery.

To come across as more well-rounded and erudite, read as much as you can and practice conveying what you have read to others. You need to learn to talk about exciting, provocative, interesting things and stay away from boring topics, such as your buddies, your favorite sports team, or the weather. What topics do most hotties find exciting? Talk about places you traveled or plan on traveling to, the latest movie or book that you have enjoyed, concerts you have been to, interesting people you've met, or the latest events in the media.

However, beware not to dominate the conversation or drone on for too long about a topic that is too complex for a woman you are trying to impress (especially if she is "the cognitively challenged beauty"). We tend to prefer mates who match our intelligence or are slightly above us. Coming across as much more intelligent than she is will be a sure turnoff to a woman, as that will make her feel inadequate. Remember, similarity in personality traits trumps everything else[31] (more on this below).

Ways of Displaying Your Intelligence

HIT	MISS
Mentioning interesting facts	Reciting endless facts
Explaining something to her	Talking down to her
Knowing a bit about everything	Arguing about everything

SPONTANEITY/RISK TAKING—YOUR BAD-BOY SIDE

As much as women value stability, always being predictable spells boredom. Our brains are prewired to dismiss boring, banal, mundane, and routine information. Being overly proper and prim, rigid and "by the book," or insisting on her always being punctual will bore your woman and eventually cause her to lose interest. Being spontaneous, on the other hand, is an antithesis to boredom—women love mysterious men who surprise them and constantly keep them guessing.

Risk taking is related to spontaneity. This is the reason why so many beautiful women end up with "bad boys"—because they are daredevils. In fact, the most frequent categories of men that such women end up with are rock stars or athletes—and what these men have in common is the sensation-seeking, risk-taking traits. Why do you think James Bond is so popular? A sure way to turn off your date is to be boring or to always play it safe. I once went out on a double date with a handsome doctor. We went to Six Flags Great Adventure, and I wanted to go on the greatest roller coaster there. Although he reluctantly agreed, he kept his eyes closed the entire time and his hands clenched on the safety bar. Needless to say, it was an instant turnoff for me!

CREATE CHARACTER AMBIGUITY

If some of the qualities described above appear to contradict one another, it is because they are indeed somewhat contrary. Strong yet sensitive, courageous yet kind, reliable yet spontaneous—combining contradictory qualities adds character ambiguity, which creates depth and mystery, surprise and tension. According to Robert Greene, "The key to both attracting and holding attention is to radiate mystery."[32] You will become a riddle she will yearn to solve.

Tip from the Scoring Experts *George Gordon Byron, known as Lord Byron, was a seducer of the brooding "bad boy" school. As Lady Caroline Lamb, one of his earliest conquests, put it, the author of "Don Juan" was "mad—bad—and dangerous to know." His most famous technique was the "underlook," lowering and tilting his head slightly, then looking upward at a woman. Furthermore, his ill-fitting clothes, fidgety movements, and limp gave women the impression of vulnerability, which appealed to their care-taking instincts. This combination of danger and vulnerability has universal appeal to women even today.*

TIP # 7: Develop personality traits that appeal to women by striving to be:

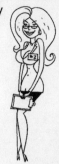

- Confident

- Kind

- Smart

- Funny

- Ambitious

- Cool

- Courteous

- Independent

- Spontaneous

Mix these up to create character ambiguity. ✦

Seven

Beyond the Bars:
Locating Your Fox's Lair

I do not approach her, I merely skirt the periphery of her existence ... This is the first web into which she must be spun ... Presumably our repeated encounters are clearly noticeable to her; presumably she does perceive that on her horizon a new planet has loomed, which in its course has encroached disturbingly upon hers in a curiously undisturbing way, but she has no inkling of the law underlying this movement ... Before I begin my attack, I must first become acquainted with her and her whole mental state.

—Søren Kierkegaard, *The Seducer's Diary*

I go from stool to stool in singles bars hoping to get lucky, but there's never any gum under any of them. —Emo Phillips

Many men complain that they don't like to go to clubs and aren't invited to many parties and therefore have difficulty finding places to meet women. This, though, just shows a lack of imagination. There are literally millions of really attractive women out there, and they don't stay home all day long pining away for Mr. Right.

They go out and do things; if you can think of what they do, you can put yourself in their field of view. You might find that they are as close as "next door"—or at least the mall a few blocks away.

In fact, you are most likely to meet the woman of your dreams if you are brought into regular contact with her through simple physical proximity (which social psychologists call *propinquity*). Through these encounters, the other person becomes someone who is recognized, no longer a total stranger, and a human being (and women in particular are always more comfortable around those they have seen before than they are with total strangers). Many of the hotties I interviewed expressed a clear preference for meeting a guy through such casual encounters created by propinquity. In addition, it is well known in social psychology that repeated exposure to almost any strange stimulus leads to an increasingly positive evaluation of that stimulus.[33] Advertising capitalizes on our tendency to respond favorably to familiar images, flooding us with repetitions of brand names, products, and electoral candidates. Thus, if you continually run into the woman of your dreams on campus, in a gym, or at the dry cleaners (accidentally, or perhaps not quite so), she is more likely to respond positively to you when you finally say hello than she would if you were a total stranger approaching her in a nightclub. Robert Greene recommends to "arrange an occasional 'chance' encounter, as if you and your target were destined to become acquainted—nothing is more seductive than a sense of destiny."[34]

▶ *Propinquity, or physical proximity, brings people together through a series of casual, accidental contacts.*

Sometimes propinquity readily presents itself, such as when a hot daughter of your local pizza shop owner serendipitously starts working for her dad during her summer vacation. All you need to do is casually greet her a few times before asking her to join you for a drink—you will look like a comfortably familiar figure. But propinquity can also be created, and those guys who have internal locus of control are out there actively concocting it. To create propinquity you have to find out her natural habitats (or hangouts, if you prefer) and make sure you become a regular part of that habitat. Think of what your prototypical woman is like and where she would be likely to spend her time. If you like women with athletic builds, you would expect them to spend time in gyms, tennis courts, skating rinks, or other athletic venues. If you like hot models, you need to frequent beauty salons, nail parlors, tanning places, and designer clothing stores. If your interests run to the more bookish type of beauty, then think Borders or Barnes & Noble, libraries, college campuses, or museums. (If you were looking for me, you'd more likely find me at Borders or the Museum of Natural History in New York City than in any nightclub.) If the next movie starlet is your ideal, your best bet is to check out acting classes, local theater groups, or auditions for *American Idol* or one of the other reality shows. Whatever you like in a woman, you can probably think of a place she would go.

While being a visitor to one of these habitats creates good opportunities for encountering these women, being a provider of that habitat is even better. For example, working out in the same gym with a hottie gives you some chances of meeting her, but being a fitness instructor increases your chances. The same goes for a shopper at the same store versus a sales manager there. A number of my centerfold friends married their hair stylists and makeup artists—these were people they saw regularly who made them feel great! If you have talent and time, become a specialist in an area that hot women are drawn to: fitness instructor, nutrition expert, yoga trainer, life coach, acting teacher, massage therapist. Any place that offers "beautification" services for women is a fine place to meet the hotties. For example, I regularly go to the Body Contouring Center, where I get endermology to combat cellulite, as well as facials, laser treatments, and other services. That place is always replete with attractive women, and the owner, a former landscaper, is married to a hot Brazilian woman whom he met at the endermology course. Such jobs have nice "fringe benefits" too. My endermology guy spends half his days removing pubic hair and massaging the torsos of one hot woman after another!

Indeed, cellulite is the bane of any model and is the number-one worry most hot women have about their bodies. It is a condition that affects just about every woman above the age of eighteen, and so it is everywhere. Just Google your hometown or state and any of the following terms: *cellulite reduction, endermology, velasmooth,* or *ioniethermie.* These terms might sound like Greek to you now, but trust me, every woman who has ever appeared in movies, on TV, or in men's magazines knows these terms intimately. When you find the places that offer these procedures, park yourself in front and wait for the bevies of beauties to appear. A line like "How come you come here? You don't have a spot of cellulite on you" is likely to be a winner in this locale. The point is, be creative in putting yourself near the kind of women you would like to meet and let propinquity play its game.

▶ *You can create propinquity by hanging out at your prototype's natural habitats.*

In fact, many hot women are reluctant to meet guys who are not familiar to them through propinquity. Penthouse Pet Brea Lynn says, "I don't give out my number to people I don't know, so unless I have seen him around, or he knows a friend, it's a no go." She met her boyfriends at school, parties, and through work. Similarly, Penthouse Pet Erica Ellyson met a few of the men she dated through track and at school. Another Pet, Krista Ayne, met the men she dated at movie and television show sets and parties. Julie Strain ended up going out with the men at comic book stores and clubs. She also hooked up with a kid from the gym—she even confessed to crashing a wedding to hook up with him. "It was the greatest affair of my life, I ended up making out with him in the mud in the pond!"

For another example, my sister met her current boyfriend at the Tae-Kwon-Do school—he was one of the instructors. "At first I did not even notice him. He was certainly not my type—too short, too young—but one day his skillful martial arts move caught my eye, and the more I watched him fight, the more turned on I became." He became her personal martial arts trainer, and eventually she discovered that he was an attentive and caring person, and a great lover in bed. "If he had approached me in a nightclub, I would never have given him the time of day. But martial arts has brought us together."

Sporting events and activities often attract the best in feminine pulchritude. Auto races, ski resorts, beaches, and horse shows sport crowds of single women; even team sporting events will elicit some hot groupies hoping to hook up with one of the athletes. Most of them won't succeed at that, so they are easy pickings for a guy who knows his sports and can mix with the jock crowd. Rock and pop concerts are great places to meet really hot women, as many models love the rock star image. My friend Penthouse Pet Krista Ayne loves men with Mohawk haircuts and rock group tattoos, so if that's your style, save up for some concert tickets.

Combining hobbies with potential dating opportunities is a great way to meet women while enriching yourself, thus making yourself more interesting to women. Try taking a photography or drama class, go to an art gallery opening or an arts and crafts class, or take up aerobics or ballroom dancing. Chances are you will be one of very few guys surrounded by excited, sexy women. Popular Playmate Barbara Moore became a ballroom dancing champion after taking it up as a hobby. One of our acquaintances (who is a pharmaceutical salesman) has a sexy hobby—he writes movie scripts, which he hopes to sell one day to a Hollywood studio. Although it may sound like a pipe dream, his ambition and lofty dreams are extremely appealing to hot women, and he picks up a ton of them by mentioning his scripts and even auditioning them for his potential films. What beautiful woman doesn't want to star in a movie?

Any place where men and money congregate, you will find gorgeous women. Casinos, racetracks, cocktail lounges, restaurants like Hooters, sports bars, and even stores and restaurants in the vicinity are all possible "hot spots." Any business where appearances count are also havens for hot chicks. Plastic surgery doctors' and cosmetic dentists' offices invariably have stunning receptionists. Fashion, design, and cosmetology schools turn out pretty students, as well as babes looking for free or discount services by serving as subjects for these students. Art schools and photography studios likewise employ sexy models. To tap these markets, hang out at nearby restaurants and coffee shops during lunch hour or happy hour and watch the birds flock in.

Believe it or not, many model types are into the occult arts, from astrology and handwriting analysis to tarot card reading and palmistry. New age stores, popular psychics, astrology classes or séances might net you a hot—if slightly daft—model or two. Just knowing a few bits of astrology will get you in the door with a lot of women, so even if you think it is sheer nonsense, it doesn't hurt to bone up on this stuff. And if you can talk triangles, pyramids, Kabbalah and Ouija boards, you will be ready to score with one of these mystic-minded maidens.

Another great place to meet women is your neighborhood coffee shop. In fact, recent surveys of online dating services say that the coffee shop is the favorite for 90 percent of those surveyed. It's also a pretty inexpensive way to spend a half hour or more meeting someone for the first time.

Malls are America's meeting places, and they are probably the easiest places to pick up hot women. Concentrate on trendy clothing and shoe stores, as both the women who work there and those who shop there are likely to be first rate. In the fancier department stores, like Bloomingdale's, Neiman Marcus, and Saks, check out the jewelry, cosmetic, perfume, and personal care counters, or the Sephora cosmetics stores, where women spend literally hours trying on makeup and skin care items. The clerks at these places are not only lookers but they are also required to be nice to their potential customers. Such cuties are easy to practice your pickup lines on. There are always great opportunities to give her and her customers compliments on their clothes, shoes, jewelry, or whatever they are buying—or to get their opinions on the gift you are thinking of buying "for your sister." An absolutely foolproof pickup moment occurs if the girl asks you for your opinion on an outfit she is considering buying. A line like "You would look great in a potato sack, but that outfit is definitely hot on you" might get you more than her phone number before the night is through.

Malls are valuable for another reason: you can tailor your targets by their shopping habits. Do you dig cute, petite types? There are stores with special departments for petites, where every woman there will fit your image. Do you like the outdoorsy types? Eddie Bauer shops and Abercrombie & Fitch are the places you want to frequent. If you love stripper types or glamour models, spend a lot of time in lingerie stores. If you like more bohemian honeys, try Pier 1, The Nature Company, and Anthropologie stores. In short, you can be very selective in choosing the scene of your hunt, such that your targets are much more likely to be on your love maps. Moreover, there is not a single beautiful woman I've ever met who doesn't like shopping, so your chances of meeting the "best of the best" are always high in those stores catering to women.

Hotel lounge bars, especially in cities known for modeling shoots, like L.A., Las Vegas, Chicago, Miami, or New York, will be where you will find the traveling glamour girl, as well as the smart businesswoman. Flown in for a shoot, which is usually finished by dark, or attending a meeting or convention, these women are often looking for a little fun, so they are more than usually approachable in this venue. I've been in this "bored in my hotel after a shoot" stage myself, especially after my nerve-wracking first nude shoot for *Playboy*—and guess what? The hotel doorman was the only one I could find to play with that night!

Another venue for meeting hot women is trade shows and conventions. Trade shows, from electronics conventions to liquor, cigar, or car shows, are full of models hired to draw attention to the company's booths. If you have a professional opportunity to attend trade shows, by all means do so. The only exceptions to this rule are conventions specifically designed for models to meet their fans, such as Glamourcons, AdultCons, and AVN. You are not likely to be as successful approaching models at this type of convention, as they are likely to lump you in the mere "fan" category, automatically disregarding you as "unsuitable" for dating. Your best approach in this kind of setting is to hang out at the bar after the show and wait to see if some of the models show up (without the boyfriend bodyguard). A number of my male friends have ended up scoring with models after Glamourcons simply by buying them drinks after the show. Plus, these kinds of shows are great places to practice talking to top models. Because they are there specifically to meet their fans, they will always talk to you; and as one guy put it, "If I am going to be rejected, I'd rather start at the top and be turned down by the hottest woman on the planet." (I thought that was a cute line—it's too bad he was off my love map.)

In the same vein, avoid approaching hot women in strip clubs. They are usually feeling vulnerable, and their focus is to make money there. They tend to have a cynical view toward men that attend adult establishments, viewing them as "losers." You will have a better chance of hooking up with one of the dancers if you moonlight there as a bouncer or a DJ. In fact, I know a radio host who does a night shift as a DJ at strip clubs and who has absolutely no problem getting laid there.

▸ *Always be ready to seize a serendipitous encounter with a sexy woman.*

Besides actively seeking out opportunities to meet hot women, you need to be on the lookout for serendipitous encounters. In fact, once you develop the self-confidence to approach women, you will realize that the opportunities are actually everywhere. Have you heard the expression "luck favors the prepared mind"? You have to be prepared to meet the women of your dreams. Look for opportunities to be helpful to a damsel in distress. If she looks lost, offer her directions and tell her you happen to be going that way. Carry a large umbrella with you on days when there is a chance of rain, and look for a beauty who forgot to check the weather forecast— then offer to walk her under yours wherever it is she is going. In fact, this is exactly how my father met my beautiful mother (who was also twenty years his junior). Like many prissy women, I hate self-service gas stations and always welcome a chivalrous guy who offers to pump the gas for me.

Finally, there are the old standbys: get your sister, your buddy, a coworker, or anyone who knows a woman you think is hot to introduce you to her. While you might not trust your little sis to pick out women you might like to date, there is no harm in taking advantage of the situation if you spot her talking to that babe you've just been dying to meet. Sometimes, you can even work out a deal with a trusted female friend. I know a guy who used to go to bars with a girl who was only a friend; they each tried to line up members of the opposite sex for each other—a mutual "wingman/ wingwoman" gig! He said this was quite successful, as there was nothing better than having an attractive woman sing your praises to another woman. These days, in some cities, there are women who act as "wingwomen" for a fee, escorting you and trying to steer your choices your way.

So the world is your oyster when it comes to meeting hot women. They are all over; you only need to think where your particular type of chick is most likely to be found, and then put yourself in her path.

TIP #8: To meet hot women: Create propinquity (proximity + opportunity) by frequenting their hangouts. ✦

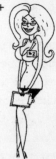

Top 10 Most Unusual Places to Meet Women

10. Clothing or shoe stores. Every woman loves to shop for apparel and footwear; if you hang out—or better yet, get a job as a salesman—in one of these shops, you will spot lots of babes in their favorite habitat. You can even pick your type of woman by specializing in the petite department, the sportswear section, or one of the other specialty shops. Shoe stores are especially convenient if you have a foot fetish—by watching them try on shoes you can eliminate those with the ugly bunions and hammertoes right away. One surefire pickup technique: watch that cute chick handle that expensive dress and reluctantly put it back; then suggest that she try it on anyway. When she does, shower her with praise for how it looks on her and insist on buying it for her! Remember, the quickest way to a woman's heart is through her wardrobe.

9. Self-improvement classes. Arts and crafts, cooking, piano, yoga, ballroom dancing, and aerobics will all yield some good candidates. Mixed-sex karate is a great class—you get a chance to feel her up before asking her out. Traffic ticket school classes make another great place to meet sensation-seeking, speed-loving females. Just pick a quality you want in a chick, and there's probably a class to find her in.

8. Casinos. Break your piggy bank, bring spare change, and offer it to the frustrated slot machine addict. If she loses, she'll be depressed (but not as depressed as she would be if it were her money), if she wins, she'll be elated—either way, anxiety and extreme emotions lead to affiliative behavior (magnifying your chances of getting laid).

7. Estate sales, garage sales, and flea markets. If you are looking for a thrift-conscious female and not a high-maintenance wallet-drainer, go to these venues regularly, or better yet, organize one yourself. If you are recently divorced, it is the perfect way to advertise your availability by getting rid of your ex's stuff. Develop an expertise in a category of stuff, like imitation Tiffany lamps or early Barbie dolls. Then wait until a hot one comes along and show her how she can get the item for a "steal." Next to a new dress, there is nothing like a bargain to put a woman in the mood.

6. Spas and salons. If you have a vain bone, capitalize on it. Get regular manicures, pedicures, and hair treatments at a women's salon. Chat up the manicurist or hairdresser—they usually know which of their regulars are single and looking. Keep your eyes open, as you never know when that hair dryer is going to reveal Princess Charming in curlers. And while you're there, get your genital area waxed—it feels great, and it will carry the additional bonus of making your penis appear larger!

5. Male review shows. If you have the body for it, become a Chippendales dancer! If you don't, moonlight there as a bouncer. Plenty of booze + nearly naked men + horny women = can't miss!

4. Soup kitchens. Up your philanthropist score by becoming a volunteer at a homeless shelter or a hospice. The women that work there are naturally giving, caring, and friendly even to the scruffiest of men. And kindness is one of the qualities women most look for in a male. Be sure to have a good sob story handy, about the times you were "down on your luck" and now want to "pay back" the community. Next thing you know, you'll be enjoying soup in her kitchen.

3. Support groups. Whether it be Alcoholics Anonymous, Shopaholics Anonymous, or a Sexual Addiction support group, group therapy is one of the best ways to create instant rapport. Misery loves company. Mmmm. Did I say "Sexual Addiction support group"? I think I need to investigate that one personally.

2. ESL classes. If you enjoy sultry South Americans or high-cheekboned Eastern Europeans, volunteer as a TA at an English-as-a-second-language course. You know how those tall, willowy blondes need special help with their language lessons! Then, too, these babes need advice on how to get along in American culture; and who are they likely to ask but their kindly teacher? Besides, nothing makes these foreign hotties hornier than a desire for a green card!

1. Meetings or conventions of women's associations. Contrary to your instinctual aversion to women's lib, National Organization of Women meetings are the perfect breeding ground for available, horny women. Other groups to frequent: pro-choice groups and my absolute favorite, the Pro-Porn Feminists. So bone up on your feminist rhetoric, remembering that liberated women are much more likely to cast away outdated notions of courtship and chivalry, letting you be the male chauvinist pig you really are. You won't have to worry about opening the door for her or paying for her dinner, and you just might get laid on the first date!

Eight

Swaggers and Smiles:
Catching Her Eye . . . and Keeping It

Glances are the heavy artillery of the flirt: everything can be conveyed in a look, yet that look can always be denied, for it cannot be quoted word for word. —STENDHAL

Now that you have located your beautiful babe and see her seated in Starbucks enjoying a grande Mocha Frappuccino, you are ready to make your move. You have conquered your initial fears about talking to women; you have practiced on less-attractive women to try out your skills; you have honed and toned your body at the gym, salons, and barbershop; and you are wearing your best girl-getting outfit. You are ready for the big score, and your target is at hand.

GETTING NOTICED

Your first and most important task is getting her attention. This is not a simple matter, as you can easily get her attention by jumping up and down, but it would crash your program if you used such obvious means. You need to have her pick you out of the background of customers, employees, and other people passing by; you want her to focus her awareness on you. Moreover, you want her to have a positive impression from that first awareness. This is the critical moment—and not the pickup line you might have practiced. If you handle this first impression right, you can say anything and she will listen with interest. Why is this so?

When we find ourselves surrounded by strangers, we make a quick mental decision as to whom we will pay attention to and whom we will ignore. This automatic mental screening response is known as *cognitive disregard*. Once disregarded, you might as well not exist, as far as the screener is concerned. In social situations, a woman's eyes sweep the crowd and she subconsciously eliminates in this way all but those who meet her standards. This mental exclusion process is based on easily observable characteristics, such as age, posture, physique, gait, and clothing. Once a person is disregarded as "unsuitable," "uninteresting," or "not my type," he becomes effectively invisible. Only after this initial exclusion process do we decide who we like among the remaining individuals.

That's why your first effort should be to make sure you are not eliminated from her consideration. How do you accomplish that? Obviously, an attractive appearance, good physique, and stylish clothing matter (as described above). However, your appearance and physique are not nearly as important as your overall demeanor. The way you use your body, your expressions, and your behavior in her hearing or vision can set you apart from the crowd. This is what will make or break your approach; the key to remaining in her visual field is to behave like an alpha male—a dominant, confident guy. How do you do that?

1. Project Dominance

It may go back to the days of the tribe or cave society in prehistoric times, but women are instinctively attracted to the dominant male. Research confirms what we know at gut level: males who behave in a dominant, extraverted way are always rated as more attractive than those whose behavior is relatively introverted or submissive. What is perceived as dominant behavior?

Expressive, gregarious guys who keep their heads high, speak with authority, maintain an upright posture, thrust their chests, take up a lot of space, and gesture a lot are perceived as more dominant and, therefore, attractive. Anthropologist Helen Fisher calls this type of behavior "looming," or attempting to look big. Behaviors like stirring his drink with his entire arm, stretching his arms back, and pivoting his feet outward would fall in the looming category. Quiet guys who look down, stoop, and frequently nod their heads in agreement when communicating with other males are seen as less attractive.

How you talk to the salesclerk or the friend you are with is going to register with that honey sipping her Frappuccino at the next table. So keep your voice firm and authoritative, show that you know what you want, be friendly and joke if appropriate, and let everyone around you know that you are simply brimming with self-confidence and self-assurance. Act like you own the place!

Ways to Project Dominance

HIT	MISS
Being gregarious	Being a loudmouth
Taking up space	Taking up the entire space
Looming	Overpowering

2. Create a Genuine Smile

Your smile is your most important tool for keeping in her field of vision. More centerfolds name "smiles" as the thing that first attracts them to men—more than any other action or behavior. They are not alone. Research has consistently shown that people of all ages, sexes, and cultures are attracted to smiles.

However, there is a big difference between genuine smiles and fake or "managed" smiles. Have you ever been fooled by the smile of a flight attendant who tells you "Have a great day!" but really means "Get the hell out-a-here so that I can go home!"? Most of the time you can tell she is faking that smile; indeed, psychologists call the fake smile a "Pan American smile" after the flight attendants on that now-defunct airline. It is rare that adults, at least, are fooled by insincere or faked smiles, because only the sides of the mouth are used, and none of the smile appears in or around the eyes. Moreover, to fake a smile you have to engage in what behavioral scientists call "emotional labor," the process of displaying one type of emotion while feeling another, and it is actually known to be very taxing on an individual over time. So if you are feeling apprehensive or nervous while trying to smile at a hot girl, your smile is likely to turn out managed and artificial.

On the other hand, when you smile spontaneously, your whole face, particularly the eyes, smile. The genuine smile (known in psychological literature as the Duchenne smile, in honor of the dude who first described it) involves the specific muscles near the eye. These muscles pull the facial skin into the "crinkly" pattern at the corners of each eye, cause the droop in the eyelid toward the temple, and pull the cheeks and corners of the mouth upward (rather than sideways as in the Pan Am smile). The Duchenne smile is accompanied by increased activity in the left prefrontal cortex, known to be the seat of positive emotions. Everybody interprets this as being spontaneous and reflecting underlying positive feelings. And when you put this kind of smile on, you automatically activate your pleasure centers, making yourself look and feel happy. So this is what you want your woman to see when she looks up at you.

The secret to creating a genuine Duchenne smile is thinking positive thoughts or envisioning a pleasant scene or outcome. That shouldn't be hard, since your target is, by definition, a hot-looking woman. That pleasant vista should always elicit a genuine Duch-

enne; and in your new, confident persona, you can be thinking of
how much fun you are going to have with her to keep that smile
going even when you are not looking at her. Actually, anything that
pleases you or makes you laugh could be floating through your
mind as you "survey" the scene and prepare to make your move,
so keep smiling frequently—and always when you look her way!

Ways to Project a Genuine Smile

HIT	MISS
Think of something happy	Think of screwing her
Smile when you look at her	Grin the entire time
Laugh	Giggle

3. Watch Your Body Language

It is very important to watch your body language while you are
moving in on a hot woman. Your body language will reveal much
about your emotional state. If you are slouching, fidgeting, biting
your lip, or making a lot of extraneous movements—especially
ones in which a particular body part does something to another,
such as scratching or rubbing—she will interpret your behavior
as nervousness.[35] Chewing gum, biting your fingernails, or chewing on the corner of your mouth are all negative behaviors. Similarly, stiffness in your limb motions suggests discomfort and tension. Keeping your hands in your pockets or crossing your arms
may be signs of nervousness too. They also tend to suggest you are
introverted.

Instead, keep your feet well apart, toes pointing outward,
shoulders back, and chest forward. Relax your arms or hold a
drink casually. Don't be afraid to take up space and time, leaning
on a counter in the middle of the bar or standing by a table in
the center of the room—like you own the place, remember. Take

your time paying for a drink or moving across the room, and never let anyone or anything rush you. Let the crowd flow around you, rather than trying to avoid the crowd. Slow, unhurried movements show that you are supremely self-confident and don't care about the opinions of others.

4. Practice a Sexy Gait

Psychological research has shown that body movement and gait can be important clues to a person's physical state and even personality traits. In one study,[36] subjects were shown videotapes of various people walking (all they could see were shadow silhouettes). They were then asked to rate the walkers in terms of a number of traits (e.g., submissive-dominating, sexy-unsexy, timid-bold) and to rate the walkers' gaits in terms of several characteristics (e.g., amount of hip sway, knee bending, short or long strides). In addition, participants estimated the walkers' ages. Results indicated that gait was indeed a very important nonverbal clue. The gait deemed to be youthful was characterized by more hip sway, knee bending, bounce, and loose-jointedness. Persons displaying such a gait were rated as sexier, happier, and stronger physically than those showing a less youthful gait. Possession of a youthful gait (regardless of actual age) was strongly related to perception of the walkers' happiness and power.

In subsequent research, participants were shown the same videotapes, but this time they could see the walkers (not merely their silhouettes). Even with all the other array of nonverbal cues, participants' ratings of the walkers were influenced by their gait. Again, walkers with a youthful gait were rated as more powerful, sexier, and happier than those with an older gait, regardless of other cues as to real age. These findings suggest that an individual's gait is an important determinant of the impression he makes on others! So put some bounce in your step, smoothness and looseness in your body movements, and you will be perceived as a younger, sexier, and more vigorous male.

5. Mirror Her Actions

Try adopting a posture similar to hers. This is called "postural congruence," "interactional synchrony," or "mirroring." Experiments have shown that people will evaluate a person who is deliberately mirroring their postures more favorably without being consciously aware of this bias. When flirting, you can use postural mirroring to create a feeling of familiarity and harmony. So if she is crossing her hands in front of her chest, do the same; and when she takes a sip of her drink, copy her move. If you can't duplicate a movement, approximate it; if she twirls her shoulder-length curls through her fingers (my habit!), you can run your hand through your hair. Make sure you do this mirroring subtly and casually, and don't try to copy any purely feminine gestures. For example, if she starts stroking her breasts, relax. She's already hot for your bod!

6. Beware Who You Are With

Another important caveat: when you are trying to scope out a woman of your dreams, you need to be mindful whose company you are in. As cruel as it sounds, do not let your goofy-looking friend tag along. You might feel braver in the company of your nerdy buddy, but having him around is likely to hurt your chances at meeting a hottie. Social research unequivocally shows that your perceived attractiveness is affected by the appearances of your companions. To put it plainly—the way your friend looks seems to rub off on you. If you are associated with someone unattractive, you are perceived as less attractive than if you are with someone who is better looking.[37/38]

That's why you are better off having a handsome (but already taken) male acquaintance or a good-looking female friend with you. The good-looking male buddy will get you easier entrée into the group of women in which your target is hanging out, and the hot girl by your side, like the "wingwoman" mentioned above, will convince other women that you are a worthy catch. Beautiful women tend to want guys who are with other hot women because of the "equity theory," which posits that people tend to assume that the less attractive individual in the mismatched pair must be rich, powerful, wise, sexy, or famous in order to make up for his "deficiencies" in appearance. If your female companion far exceeds you in attractiveness, women are likely to explain this by imbuing you with more positive characteristics, thinking, *He must have something special to attract a woman like that.* And, of course, you do—you really know how to satisfy a woman, especially after reading this book!

TIP #9: To get the woman to notice you:

• Act in a dominant way by keeping your head high, maintaining upright posture, taking up a lot of space, and gesturing a lot

• Adopt a relaxed, youthful gait

• Smile a lot and "for real" by thinking of something positive

• Subtly imitate her movements

• Ditch your nerdy buddy ✦

Top Signs You Shouldn't Try to Approach Her

1. She is wearing a baseball cap and sunglasses

2. She is with her parents or business associates

3. She is engrossed in her book or newspaper

4. She is on her cell phone

5. She is crying or obviously upset

6. She is alone in a dark alley

7. She looks pissed off

MOVING IN

Words are only painted fire; a look is fire itself.

—MARK TWAIN

Most guys think that successful flirting depends upon coming up with the "right pickup line." The reason why guys obsess over pickup lines is in large part because they don't realize that the content of what they say is far less important than the context in which it is said, and that their nonverbal behavior plays a far larger role in making an impression on women than the cleverness of their lines. When you first meet a woman, she will base 55 percent of her initial impression on your appearance and body language, 38 percent on your style of speaking, and only 7 percent on what you actually say. Indeed, I hardly remember any of the thousands of lines I've been thrown by would-be pickups, but I vividly remember the other aspects of a man's looks and behavior that attracted me to him. The key to making a good impression is to remain cool, collected, and composed while you are talking to a hot woman. The only way to become that way is by practicing your approach with many different women. Practice makes perfect. So if you really want to flirt with a woman and entice her to go out with you, throw out those stale, stupid pickup lines and concentrate on the things that count, like those below:

1. Use Your Eyes to Make Contact

Look at her. All over. Linger anywhere you like. When she notices (and she will if you are really looking), hold her eyes with yours. . . . You'll know then and there whether she wants you or not.   —SUSIE BRIGHT

Your eyes are your primary flirting tools. Strong eye contact calls for human connection and intimacy—no wonder eyes have been termed the "windows to the soul." Humans automatically interpret a high level of eye contact from another as a sign of liking and friendliness.[39]

Famous anthropologist Helen Fisher calls this romantic gaze the "copulatory gaze." The "copulatory gaze" is an intense stare at the object of your interest, during which your pupils dilate, your eyelids drop, and then you then look away. This eye contact appears to trigger a primitive part of the human brain calling for either "approach" or "retreat" behavior. The copulatory gaze may be an evolutionary behavior embedded in our psyches, as other primates have been observed to stare deeply into each other's eyes before engaging in coitus. Try engaging a woman with your eyes by staring at her intensely for a few seconds, then dropping your eyelids and diverting your gaze. If she is interested, she will likely respond with the copulatory gaze of her own followed by a smile the next time you glance at her.

One caveat: It is important to drop your eyelids and look away after a few seconds of intense gaze because a continuous uninterrupted gaze can be interpreted as staring, which makes people nervous and tense.[40] Unlike gazing, staring can be interpreted as a sign of hostility and confrontation and often prompts a desire to retreat.[41] So avoid staring at her or scoping her body up and down (known as "elevator eyes"), as that may betray your lust and make her feel uncomfortable.

2. Use Your Face to Signal Interest

Once you make eye contact, you can signal your interest by a smile or light head nod. These are called nonverbal solicitation signals. The smile is the clearest signal; if you get a smile in return, you know you've earned a favorable reaction. A wink is also sexy, especially if you have gotten that return smile—although make sure it is a Duchenne!

If you want to grab the attention of a cute chick over on the other side of the room, you can also try the "eyebrow flash." It involves raising the eyebrows very briefly, for about one-sixth of a second, and it is used to signal recognition. One caveat: Do not use the eyebrow flash in Japan, where it has definite sexual connotations and can earn you a slap across a cheek.

3. Make the Move without Hesitating

When you have gotten her attention, fully engaged her eyes, and given her your best Duchenne smile, nod, or eyebrow flash, you will be looking for her response. She will probably avert or lower her eyes, and she might smile coyly. When she looks away, start counting! Research on flirtation shows that if she looks at you again within 45 seconds, you have caught her interest. If she is not interested, she will make an effort not to look in your direction. If she turns away, stops smiling, or purposefully avoids looking at you, drop her and look for another hottie.

Once you catch her gaze for the second time, give her a friendly, closed-mouth smile (avoid teeth baring or lecherous grins). You can also nod, wink, or give her an eyebrow flash—whichever you feel most comfortable with. Once you have signaled your interest, you must make your move. If you continue to stare without approaching her, you will betray your hesitancy, or worse, risk looking like a stalking buffoon. And the more time you allow yourself to vacillate, the more doubts will start creeping into your mind. Or worse yet, she will be approached by another Lothario. Remind yourself that "he who hesitates is lost," then banish all negative thoughts, using one of the techniques described above. Move toward her immediately!

Ways of Getting Her Attention

HIT	MISS
Gaze for a few seconds	Stare
Wink, it comes out natural	Wink, it looks like a tic
Maintain eye contact	Look her up and down
Closed-mouth genuine smile	Ear-to-ear tooth-baring grin
Nod or eyebrow flash	Wolf whistle

Signs She Is Interested

✦ *Welcoming gestures:* looking at you, glancing down, sneaking repeated glances, eyes sparkle, pupils enlarge, giving a genuine lip-corners-up smile

✦ *"Crouching" gestures:* putting her hands to her face, pointing her feet inward

✦ *Intention gestures:* rubbing her leg or arm, licking her lips

✦ *Grooming gestures:* playing with her hair, reapplying makeup, straightening clothes

✦ *Orienting gestures:* turning body toward you, angling her head, pushing breasts forward

✦ *Mirroring gestures:* holding glass the same way, leaning in the same direction

Tip from the Scoring Experts *Pablo Picasso, the famous painter noted for pioneering Cubism, was not physically attractive, but he had an alluring way of gazing at women, which led them to see him as a man of inner magnetism. His fire and drive were what attracted many mistresses to his bed—of course, a bit of artistic talent helped too.*

TIP #10: To approach her:

• Look at her intently, then lower your eyes and look away

• Gaze at her again, and see if she averts her eyes then looks again within a minute

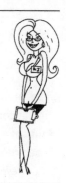

• Smile, nod, wink, or use an eyebrow flash to signal your approach

• Make the move without hesitating ✦

Myth Rebuffed: YOU MUST APPROACH A WOMAN IN THE FIRST THREE SECONDS.

This rule puts too much pressure on a guy without affording substantial benefit, although the sooner you approach her, the better. Approaching her right as you see her might look to her like a knee-jerk reaction to her sex appeal, as opposed to your response to something special about her. Giving yourself a couple of minutes to evaluate the situation (Is she with a guy? Is she in a hurry?) is always a good idea. If she is wearing a flashy outfit, you can take a moment to check it out and use it in your approach ("Love your shoes: are they Prada?" "I know the low-riders are really in now, but they can't possibly be comfortable"). If there is some outfit malfunction, you can be the helpful bystander ("Be careful, your purse is open," etc). Having said that, do not hang around her, staring and grinning. If you need some extra time to get into RIS, order a drink, make a phone call, or chat with someone else for a minute. You must, however, approach her within five to eight minutes of making intense eye contact with her to avoid appearing insecure or creepy.

Nine

Beyond Pickup Lines: Striking Up Some Sparks

A gossip is one who talks to you about others, a bore is one who talks to you about himself; and a brilliant conversationalist is one who talks to you about yourself. —LISA KIRK

Man hits on woman at bar: "Would it help if I told you how moved I was by 'The Vagina Monologues'?" —LEE LORENZ

You're walking up to where she is sitting at her table, almost finished with her Frappuccino. There is a genuine but closed-mouth smile on your face, your shoulders are straight, your gait is rolling and confident, and you're ready to meet the girl of your dreams. Now what?

There are "dating coaches" who will take two hundred to one thousand dollars from you to teach you "great pickup lines." You'd be wasting your money if you tried a single one of them on any of the centerfold models I know. Virtually all of them wrote on my questionnaires such comments as "Just be normal," "Don't try to impress," "Keep it real," "Talk to me like I was just your friend," "If you like me, say so," or words to that effect. In short, they just want you to start a conversation by making a comment. It's that simple.

How to Start a Conversation

Psychology supports the conclusion that being straightforward, "real," and relatively "friendly" is the best conversation opener. One study[42] characterized opening remarks as falling into three categories:

Cute-flippant: *Isn't it cold? Let's make some body heat.*

Innocuous: *Where are you from?*

Direct: *Hi. I like you.*

Overall, the most preferred lines were innocuous or direct, and the least preferred were cute-flippant. Women tend to be much more negative about the cute-flippant lines and more positive about innocuous lines than men were. The authors of the study went on to conclude that those who work hard to come up with an amusing line in order to make a good impression usually produce the exact opposite effect. Why do so many folks use the cute-flippant pickup lines? The authors of this study suggested that the reason these lines are common is that people, particularly men, fear rejection and defend themselves by using humor. And a small minority of women do respond positively to a clever line. I would guess that a woman who normally does not get that much attention might respond positively to a cute-flippant line, particularly if it is a flattering one such as "It must be real sweet to be your lips." Hot women, however, are unlikely to appreciate cute-flippant lines because they hear these lines all the time from obnoxious guys not afraid to approach them.

Using an innocuous line is a much safer strategy because it

doesn't offend anyone (thus protecting the guy against rejection) and increases the likelihood that a woman will respond positively. Keep in mind that adding terms of endearment such as "honey," "babe," "doll," or "sweetie" can give an innocuous line a cute-flippant undertone. A majority of hotties I interviewed expressed dislike for guys who used these terms of familiarity in their pickup lines. Although many sexy young women do not mind being called "babe," others consider it to be condescending and take offense—so use these terms at your own risk! Below are various approaches that allow you to incorporate direct, cute-flippant, and innocuous lines in the most effective way.

Remember, prepare a few questions for her to answer, and don't talk more than a minute before giving her an opening question. If you prefer more innocuous approaches over direct ones, you can benefit from carrying a few props that could be used to initiate a conversation, such as a newspaper, an umbrella, an attaché case, or a camera. A current newspaper makes a wonderful prop because you can use it to comment on the latest events or celebrity gossip, ask her help in solving a crossword puzzle, or offer to read her the horoscope. A camera is great for both direct and indirect approaches: you can tell her you are an apprentice photographer and you would love to snap a shot of her beautiful face, if she doesn't mind; if you have a digital camera, you can ask her opinion of some of the shots you have taken so far. The best way to utilize a prop is to make it consistent with your prototype—if she loves musicians, you should carry your guitar case with you any time you are out hunting for hot babes.

Express Your Interest

Although many sexy women I interviewed said they would prefer a direct approach, it is actually not the one I would recommend, unless you are experienced with meeting women or have reached the RIS. The reason women prefer the direct approach is that it is flattering, it takes the guesswork out, and it gives them full power to accept or reject a man's proposal. For that reason, a direct approach puts a guy in a more vulnerable position than an innocuous approach would. The direct approach is still better for a novice than a cute-flippant approach, because with the former a woman is unlikely to be offended, and, if she is not interested, she is most likely to politely decline, whereas a guy using a cute-flippant approach risks a rude response from a prude or a woman with little sense of sexual humor.

Here is how you could directly display your interest in meeting the Frappuccino-drinking hottie in the example above:

> *"Hi, would you mind if I sit next to you so that we could enjoy our Frappuccinos together?"*

Here's an approach that blends a direct line with a cute-flippant one:

> *"We both like Starbucks, it's a good start. Let's see if we have anything else in common. Coffee, tea, or me?"*

Compliment Her

Compliments make it obvious that you like her, but if you are a direct guy who prefers a direct approach, compliments make great opening lines, as long as you keep them tactful, safe, and neutral. Think about what made you notice this woman. Her eyes, her hair, her outfit, and her smile make your best bets. However, do not use stock phrases like "You have beautiful eyes" unless you really find her eyes beautiful. Women have an intuitive radar for a lack of candor. Instead, try to look for her unique features. For example, you can comment on her adorable freckles or her luscious hair or her beautiful manicure. A guy who compliments my French manicure always scores a point with me because I know he notices finer details and is not staring at my chest. One guy once complimented me on my long fingers. He said, "You have long fingers, you could be a hand model." I ended up talking to him for an hour—it turned out he was a food photographer.

Obviously, if you can come up with an insightful and original compliment, you will score an additional point with her. I was once wearing a polka dot dress reminiscent of the '50s in a club full of women clad in low-rider jeans, and I felt a bit out of place. I felt great when a guy came up to me and said, "I love that retro look on a woman, it reminds me of timeless Hollywood glamour. But most young girls these days just don't have the elegance to pull it off. You, on the other hand, look better than Grace Kelly." His compliment hit bull's-eye, right in the center of my vain spot—I do consider myself possessing a more refined taste than most attractive women. But if nothing seems to come to mind, don't beat yourself up trying to invent an original line. You can say something like "White looks great on you, it makes your shiny black hair stand out." If you care to brush upon the latest women's fashions, you'll have a ton of easy openers at hand for beauties, as high-maintenance women enjoy talking about fashion, clothing, and accessorizing. They spend a lot of time choosing what to wear, and they feel good in the presence of a guy with a discerning eye for haute couture who can appreciate their efforts.

Avoid complimenting obviously intimate body parts such as her breasts, or obviously fetish ones, such as her feet. Hold off on addressing her obvious sexual attributes unless she specifically invites your opinion. "You have a great ass, babe!" is a great compliment when you are naked and in bed together, but when you are still getting to know one another, it is both crude and a turnoff to most women.

Comment on the Surroundings

Whereas a direct or cute-flippant approach does work for many guys, an innocuous approach is your safest bet. How do you come up with an innocuous line? Simply make a statement relevant to the situation. You can use what is called Impersonal Interrogative Comment (IIC)—a general comment on some aspect of the event, activity, or ambience, with a rising intonation, or "isn't it?" type of ending. Here are a few examples: "This artist is talented, isn't he?" or "I wonder who picked the music for this event. It's pretty good, isn't it?" If she is not interested, her response will be short and unenthusiastic, and you can retreat without humiliation.

When you use an IIC you have to be careful not to come across as a whining complainer. A comment like "Service in this place is really slow, don't you think?" sounds like a real downer, and mentioning negative things is likely to bring her down. Another disadvantage of the IIC is that it can sound boring and it doesn't engage her in conversation. The best way to utilize an IIC is to follow it up with a cute line if she appears to be interested. You can say something like "It's cold in here, isn't it?" If she responds, "Yes, it sure is," you can then say, "But your presence can melt an iceberg."

Ask Her a Question

Another easy innocuous approach is to ask her a question. Ask her what time it is, tell her that she looks familiar, or inquire how her day is going or how she knows the host of the party. But avoid opening with a question calling for very personal information, such as "What do you do?" or "What are you thinking?" Also, avoid questions that are so nebulous that they put pressure on her to come up with a clever answer. My personal pet peeve is "What's up?" I've been asked that a million times, and I've never come up with a good response. I usually say "Nothing is up," because I hate this question—and it instantly kills any further conversation. Do not expect a woman to provide a lengthy response to a general comment like that; she is not there to entertain you. Instead, you need to actively engage her in a conversation.

Although you can start your opener with a question, your opener will sound smoother if you preface it with a comment. For example, upon hearing my accent, a lot of guys will ask me, "Where are you from?" This is an acceptable opener when approaching a girl with an accent. However, if you want to sound more erudite and worldly, you might want to guess where she is from instead. "You have a slight accent, which sounds German or Dutch. Am I right?" or "You are probably sick of hearing this, but you don't look or sound like you are originally from the U.S. Are you Eastern European (South American, etc)?" If you are drawn to foreign women, you should learn to distinguish various accents, as well as hone up your geography and linguistic skills. There is nothing more embarrassing than not knowing what she is talking about when she answers, "I am actually from Lisbon. Do you know where that is?" I have had numerous guys who got a great start by saying "I love Eastern European women, I think they are the hottest women around," but then had no idea that Kiev, my hometown, was the capital of Ukraine. Learning a couple of different words in various languages also provides for great openers and conversation extenders.

Pickup Lines You Can Get Away With

"You don't look old enough to drink." When she answers, "I am," you can respond, "Do you remember the times we could not wait to be old enough to drink legally, and now I love when I get carded!"

"Your smile lights up the room." You should use this line only if she has a nice smile. Women love to be complimented on their smiles.

"You look like you are having fun." You can follow up with "What's your story?" This line can sound upbeat and uplifting, as opposed to "You look bored" or "What's up?" which I personally dislike.

"How was your day?" If she responds "Great," you could ask her what happened during the course of her day. If she responds by saying "OK," you can probe further into what made her day not so great, empathizing in the process.

"You seem to be the kind of person I would enjoy getting to know." If she responds "Yes" or "Why?" you could say, "You look intriguing. There is a sparkle of personality and intelligence in your eyes, you are not just a pretty face."

"Do you know you look like . . . ?" If she says, "I've been told that before," ask her whether she considers that celebrity to be a good actress, a positive role model, etc.

"You look familiar." Acting like you know her from somewhere is always a good approach. It is particularly effective with models and actresses because they often seek fame and, therefore, feel very flattered when they are recognized. Glance at her, then look at her again, squinting your eyes, as if trying to remember where you met her before. You can then tell her that you must have met her before, and ask her if you look familiar to her. If her response is an unenthusiastic "No," you can just tell her, "You look just like a girl I went to school with" and move on.

Ask Her Opinion or Advice

Another good way to innocuously open a conversation is to ask for her opinion or advice on something. This works best if you haven't been exchanging glances or flirting with her beforehand and just "happen" to be standing next to her. If you are standing next to her in a deli, deciding on what to get, you can begin by musing out loud: "I wonder if I should have that tuna sandwich or the shrimp salad," then turn to her and say, "The shrimp salad looks kind of soggy, and shrimp is never good after it's been sitting around for a few days. What do you think?" This way you give her plenty of material to comment on—and most women like to express their opinions, especially when it comes to food, clothes, furniture, and other household items. A guy once picked me up in Las Vegas by asking me my opinion on a soft toy: "I have a six-year-old daughter and I wonder if I should get her a striped tiger or white one?" "A striped one," I said. "I knew you'd recommend a striped one," he responded. "Why is that?" I inquired. "Because you look like you prefer fancier rather than simpler things in life, judging by your lovely outfit," he retorted, making me smile. From there on the conversation flowed, he bought me a striped tiger, and that night we ended up in bed together. Obviously, stay away from asking her opinions on topics she is likely to be clueless or uninterested about, like "I wonder if I should get an eight-point wrench or a flat spanner, what do you think?"

Here are two examples of opening a conversation with your Frappuccino hottie by asking her opinion or advice:

• "This place does incredible business, doesn't it?" When she responds, you can show off your entrepreneurial spirit by expanding on your business idea: "I want to come up with a similar concept. What do you think of me opening a tea place with every imaginable type of tea from all over the world?" The great thing about this line is that it sounds like you are simply gathering polls concerning a potential business you want to start, rather than trying to pick her up.

• "Hey, I am debating between a raspberry Mocha or Chocolate Brownie Frappuccino. What do you think?" Once she responds, you can agree with her suggestion or say something like "You look like a chocolate lover. I love chocolate, but the brownie one might be too much. A little chocolate is actually good for us, but too much tends to clog up our arteries, and I see too many heart attacks to let that happen to me." Chances are she will love to continue this conversation—what woman doesn't like to talk about the pros and cons of chocolate? This will be your chance to show off how health-conscious you are, especially if she looks fit and has a gym bag next to her.

Make a Helpful Comment or Ask Her to Do You a Favor

Another approach is to make a helpful comment. This works especially well if she appears to be looking for something or she has a small equipment malfunction. If you see her spill her coffee, you can tell her where to get some napkins. Or if her lipstick smeared, you can point that out to her. If she is balancing her coffee in one hand and her purse in the other, you can offer to help. Another trick is to carry a pair of old keys so that you can pretend you have just found them: inquire if they are hers or if she knows anyone who they might belong to. You can then follow up with a funny story of what happened once when you lost your keys. You can also ask her to do you a small favor, e.g., watch your briefcase when you go to the bathroom.

Make a Joke and/or Tell a Funny Story

Finally, you can open by making a joke or telling a funny story. Obviously, this one works best if you are naturally witty, quick on your feet, or facile with storytelling. But don't be down on yourself if you are not—very few men are naturally witty enough to come up with spontaneously funny quips (and many of those who can are quite eccentric). If you run into your hottie in the same place on a regular basis, you can prepare a funny line or story. For example, if she tends to frequent your Starbucks, when you are next to her in line, say to her, "Where did they come up with that word *Venti* to indicate a large coffee? Last time I was here I saw a tourist browsing an English dictionary trying to translate *Venti*. He looked so confused, poor thing."

Here are some other examples of this approach, such as making a funny comment and storytelling:

• "Is the size of your drink tall, grande, or venti? I can never remember which one is which." When she responds, you can show your nonconformist spirit by making fun of the ridiculous size nomenclature: "I think these names are preposterous—why can't we call a spade a spade? Why can't I just ask for a large coffee? Do you think people actually prefer the fancy names?" Once she offers her opinion, you can show off your funny bone by feigning indignation. "I was recently in Dallas, and they have a Starbucks competitor, Seattle's Best Coffee. They went even further by calling their large-size cup grandesupremo! I guess if I want to outcompete them I should call a large cup a mega grandissimo giganto!"

Tease her while storytelling:

• "Be careful not to spill that! My attorney friend is handling a case of someone who got injured by a hot Frappuccino just like yours!" After she responds, you can comment on how ridiculously litigious our society has become, and tell her about another ridiculous lawsuit you have read about.

Remember, it is really not all that important what line you choose as long as you are comfortable with it and it suits your personality and advances the prototype you want to project. If you want to come across as an Entertainer, debate the ludicrous drink names with her; if you are an Enterpreneur type, ask her opinion about opening a similar business; if you are an Advocate, comment on how overworked the poor employees seem to be. The more openly you display your interest, the more vulnerable you make yourself to rejection—so attempt it only if you have achieved the Rejection Immunity State.

✦ ✦ ✦

Here are some approaches framed with a prototype you are trying to project. Obviously, they work best if you are actually that person—I don't recommend deceit for the purpose of picking up women, although white lies are OK as long as they are consistent with your overall values. For instance, you can approach her telling her you are looking for individuals to join your new charity. You don't have to have the charity organized yet, as long as you are the kind of person who actually engages in charity work. Otherwise, you will come across as phony and disingenuous. Within minutes, you will find out whether she is into you—and whether you will be into her as well. If she doesn't go for you, then you are probably not on her love map, but if you are, you will score big time! If you make a joke and she doesn't laugh, why would you want to hang out with a woman who would not appreciate your sense of humor? If you make an intellectual comment and she looks like you are speaking a foreign language, you will probably have to "dumb down" every time you speak to her. The greatest thing about the prototype-based approach is that it doesn't look like you are trying to pick her up at all but simply having a conversation with another human being. For these, it is best that you don't flirt or make eye contact first; just go ahead and begin speaking, as if she were familiar to you.

"The Entertainer" Being entertaining and funny is probably the easiest way to pick up women. However, unlike many pickup artists who claim that any guy could learn the art of entertaining, I don't believe that's true. Some guys are innately amusing, animated, and quick-witted, and others are not. Don't try to become one if you are not! If you do have a funny bone, use it! You can come up to her and tell her that you are writing a comedy routine—you are trying to be a stand-up comedian and you want to see what she thinks of it. I was once picked up by a guy who had this ventriloquist sock puppet in his hand—which made the most obnoxious sexual innuendos toward me while his owner feigned embarrassed indignation at its behavior. It was hilarious! Another guy got my attention when he made my cell phone "disappear" as part of his magic routine.

"The Writer" The greatest thing about writers is that they are always collecting information for their work. You can approach her by telling her you are collecting female opinions for a book you will be proposing to your book agent or an article for a local newspaper. If you like poetry (I adore it), you can write a few different poems, scribble them on pieces of paper, and carry them in your pocket. If you see a hot woman, pretend that you have just composed it and give it to her. You can also say that you are working on a script for a TV show or a movie deal and need a female opinion on the matter. I have a friend who picks up most women that way, by mentioning that he is writing a movie script—and he has been actually writing it for the past ten years!

"The Philanthropist" Demonstrate some random acts of kindness in front of her. Make up a Found Puppy sheet and carry it with you. When you see a hot woman, give it to her and ask her to post it in her neighborhood. Tell her you found a puppy and now you are looking for its owner. Or put together an online charity or cause, and then solicit hot women to help you out with it. Tell her your beloved niece almost died from anorexia, and you are collecting signatures from women to ban really skinny models from runways. Would she mind signing it if you e-mailed it to her?

"The Psychic" Spill some coffee on a napkin and fold it together, making something resembling a Rorschach test. Lean over to her and ask, "What do you think this looks like?" When she responds, say, "You know what Freud would say about it?" Similarly, you can use palmistry, reading tea leaves or coffee grounds, astrology, handwriting analysis, and other fortune-telling tricks to get her to open up. Open your newspaper and look over the horoscope section, then turn to her and say, "My horoscope is totally on point today. It says I will meet an impressive person. You want to see what yours says?" This approach is likely to work with most hot women because they love fortune-telling (except me, as I am totally not into it!).

"The Entrepreneur" This works well if you walk in holding a newspaper. Pretend to look it over, then say to her, "I am thinking of investing in a Planet Beach franchise. Do you think it would make money around here? Do women still go to tanning salons a lot?" Or you can ask her to watch your attaché case as you head to the bathroom. You can say something like, "Do you mind watching my briefcase for a minute? I am tired of lugging it around all day, but it's full of important business documents for a major deal."

"The Defender" Have your buddy pretend to be an obnoxious jerk who is annoying her or disturbing her peace. You come and rescue her from him, or simply reprimand him on his disorderly conduct. Or you can tell her to watch her purse because you recently had to chase down a robber who snatched an old woman's purse. Obviously, this works best if you are actually a cop or a bodyguard.

"The Athlete" Approach a hot woman and tell her that you work for a health club and they are recruiting fit people by giving out free memberships. Ask her if she is interested in one, and if she is, get her number so that you can contact her with all the necessary info later. This obviously works best if you not only belong to a gym but also do some personal training there—this way you can weasel some free memberships out of your club manager.

"The Intellectual" Make an intellectual comment on some aspect of the environment. If she is drinking red wine, lean over and say to her, "Red wine has the most antioxidants of any alcoholic beverage out there. And you look like you get plenty of antioxidants—your skin is glowing!" You can also pull out your newspaper and begin doing a crossword puzzle, then ask her to help you out with it (just pick the easiest entry).

"The Artist" Compliment her on her unique beauty, then tell her you would like to paint her or photograph her sometime for your online portfolio. Or you can simply draw a portrait and hand it to her, telling her she inspired you. Sign it on the back and include your e-mail address. You can even tell her that you are looking for a muse, and, if she is interested, you can give her your information. If you are more of The Entertainer than The Artist, draw a silly stick figure and hand it to her, telling her that she really inspired your creative juices. You will get a smile out of most women.

TIP #11: To open a conversation:

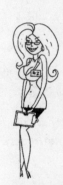

- Ask for her advice

- Inquire her opinion

- Make a helpful comment

- Make a funny/teasing comment

- Compliment her

- Ask her to do you a favor

- Tell her a funny story ✦

Conversation Openers

HIT	MISS
How was your day?	What's going on?
You look happy, what's your story?	Whass up?
Watch out, your purse is open.	What is your name?
Hi, have we met before somewhere?	Hi, my name is Bill.
Can't decide what I feel like ordering.	Can I buy you a drink?
You look radiant (if she does).	You look bored.
This place is pretty entertaining.	This place is boring, isn't it?
You look like you're enjoying yourself.	Having fun yet?
That drink/dessert is very hot/messy.	That drink/dessert has too many calories.

Ten

Buzzwords and Attitude Similarity: Nailing Her Number

Censure the things she censures,
Endorse her endorsements, echo her every word,
Pro or con, and laugh whenever she laughs; remember,
If she weeps, to weep too: take your cue
From her every expression. . . .   —OVID, *The Art of Love*

Birds are taken with pipes that imitate their own voices and men with those sayings that are most agreeable to their own opinions.
                                                        —SAMUEL BUTLER

HOW TO EXTEND A CONVERSATION

Some guys get "stuck" after the initial approach, trying too hard to come up with something clever to say next. Guys, don't worry—unless you say something demeaning or offensive to her, it won't make a difference, because she is not paying much attention to what you are saying. Most of the time she knows that you are just looking for an excuse to talk to her. What she is doing is sizing you up—your dress, your mannerisms, and your demeanor. If you remain cool, collected, in control, and, most important, unaffected by her beauty, she is likely to keep on talking to you.

Attend to Buzzwords or "Word Hooks"

Most guys don't know how to continue the conversation after the first few opening lines. The biggest faux pas they make is to follow one question with another. The conversation should flow naturally, like a tennis match, with both parties exchanging questions and comments. You can use a compliment as a conversation extender. If she offers her opinion on something, you can say something like "You know a lot about this subject" or "I like that you are candid and not afraid to speak your mind," "You are not only beautiful but also intelligent," "You have an infectious smile."

If she is reserved and does not ask you any questions, you need to be prepared to reflect or comment on her answers, or tell her some stories or disclose a bit of personal information to get her to open up. But resist the temptation to ask her a ton of factual questions—do not sound like you are interviewing her for a job. Nothing annoys me more than a guy who says, "Where are you from?" followed by "How long have you been in the U.S.?" followed by "How do you like it here?" followed by "Do you still have family over there?" followed by "Have you been back since?"

Believe it or not, this feels like a KGB interrogation to me! It makes me feel like an alien who has just landed on planet Earth. Never, ever attempt this line of questioning with a woman you have just met, or you will lose any chance of hooking up with her. This is particularly irritating to a woman who is not native to the U.S.— she has been asked the same annoying questions over and over again since she came here. More than anything, many of these women want to fit in and be the all-American girl, and this kind of crude interrogation makes them feel uncomfortable. What you want to do is use her answers as your point of reference to delve deeper into her soul rather than to dig all around on the superficial ground. The key is to be looking for buzzwords, or words that you can use as hooks to get the conversation going or to get her to open up more. For example:

YOU: How do you like this gym? (Don't start with "Where are you from?")

ME: It's OK. It's kind of crowded. (*Crowded* is your "word hook"; use it to continue the conversation.)

YOU: I am like you, I don't like big crowds. Do you know any health food stores around here? (You point out our similarity by saying "I am like you.")

ME: I don't know this area very well, I am not from here originally. (*Not from here* is your word hook.)

YOU: I have noticed a barely perceptible accent. It's very alluring. You weren't born in the U.S., right?

ME: No, I was born in Kiev, Ukraine. (*Ukraine* and *Kiev* are your buzzwords.)

YOU: I love Chicken Kiev! And Ukraine used to be part of the USSR, right? Soviet women used to be portrayed as these fat, portly women. Meanwhile, you are the hottest import we have ever gotten! You probably had a lot of propaganda about the Evil Americans, too?

ME: Yup, we did. As a matter of fact, I was really scared to come here as a student because of all the negative propaganda. (*Scared* is your buzzword.)

YOU: That is scary to move here from a different country. It must have been tough! I admire your courage. I am not sure I could have done it. How did you deal with your fear?

Now the conversation is delving deeper—from mere facts into feelings, the beginning of intimate exchange—which is the key to her heart and her bedroom.

Create a Sense of Intimacy

Have you ever gotten the feeling when talking with a stranger that you have known this person for a long time? You can actually create that sort of feeling by utilizing the right language. When people first meet, they tend to engage in small talk, exchanging pleasantries, clichés, facts, and banalities. As the relationship progresses, they tend to delve into more personal discussions and begin to share feelings with each other. You can fool her brain into believing that you are her long-lost soul mate by skipping the superficial talk and getting more personal. Sharing beliefs and feelings creates a sense of closeness and intimacy, and you don't have to get all mushy and melodramatic. Instead of impersonal "What would you like to drink," ask her "I love this drink, wanna try it?" Or comment on your feelings about some aspects of the environment while attempting to elicit her feelings. For example, you can say, "The beat of this song really gets me going. Do you like this performer?" If she responds that she does or that she prefers another one, you can express your agreement by saying, "I am with you on that one." Another way of upping the conversational intimacy level is by using "we" statements. Tell the bartender that "we really love that drink," or the host of the party that "we really love your place." If you are attending a boring lecture together, whisper to her on how "we've got to survive ten more minutes."

Use Her Name Often

Another way to reinforce a feeling of intimacy is to address her by her name frequently while conversing with her. Once she introduces herself, make sure to remember her name. Ask her what her family and friends call her, and use that name. If you happen to forget her name, ask her, "So how do you like to be called?" or "Do you abbreviate your name?" Do not take the liberty of abbreviating her name unless she gives you specific permission to do so. I really hate being called "Vickie" or "Vic"; I prefer "Victoria" or "Vika." Once she tells you, use her name often. Most people love the sound of their own name, and for women it's particularly intoxicating.

Be an Active Listener

It is far more important to know how to listen than how to talk. Once you have engaged her in a conversation, make sure to keep her interest through appropriate facial expressions. Raising your eyebrows to display surprise, nodding to indicate agreement, and smiling to punctuate a joke help keep her attention. Do not blow it by "spacing out" and blankly staring at her chest! Make sure to follow up her statements with questions that ask What, Who, How, and Where. To get her to open up, paraphrase what she says, preferably interpreting her emotion. For example, if she says, "I had to wait half an hour to get in this club," you can respond by saying, "You must have been really frustrated waiting outside in this cold weather." This technique, called reflective listening, is what shrinks use to get their patients to open up and develop rapport; use the same technique, and before you know it, she will be on your couch! Women get really turned on by a guy who attends to and appears to understand their feelings. Before she knows what is happening, she will think you have known her forever—and she will be ready to continue that relationship!

Create Attitude Similarity

It's a common folk wisdom that "birds of a feather flock together." Since the time of Aristotle, who noted that we tend to like people with similar attitude, it has been well-known that people respond more positively to those who agree with them and most negatively to those who disagree. Researchers have noted that as two people begin to interact, each person responds to the other on the basis of the proportion of similar attitudes expressed. The higher the proportion of similar views, the more the person is liked, and the lower the proportion of similarity, the more he is disliked. So forget about the expression "opposites attract," as decades of social science research has proven otherwise. If you want to capture the heart of your dream woman, you need to show her how similar you are to her in attitudes, beliefs, values, and life goals. Research has found that women are affected much more by attitude similarity than men are.[43] One of the reasons for this is that guys are so affected by the sight of an attractive woman's face and body that they tend to disregard everything else, including her values.

Use Reciprocal Disclosure

Finally, one of the most important aspects of verbal flirting is what psychologists call "reciprocal disclosure"—the exchange of personal information. People who disclose information about themselves are preferred to those who are unwilling to reveal much.[44] If she discloses some personal detail, you should reciprocate as soon as possible by revealing some similar information about yourself. However, avoid revealing too much about yourself too soon; instead, escalate the level of intimacy gradually. Obviously, most of the information you reveal should be positive (without being a braggadocio), although you can occasionally make a funny self-deprecating comment to give her a glimpse of your inner vulnerability. But be careful not to reveal anything too negative. Mentioning to her that you, too, tend to bite your nails, or that you are allergic to mint liquors, or that tight spaces make you claustrophobic is likely to make her feel closer to you, whereas telling her about your string of divorces or DUIs is likely to turn her off. Revealing a little foible about yourself is endearing, as it suggests honesty and sincerity, qualities that women look for in men.

Use Lighthearted Humor

Studies have shown that people who use humor in social encounters are perceived as more likeable, and that both trust and attraction increase when a lighthearted approach is used. An appropriately used, slightly risqué joke can escalate the level of intimacy—but keep the gross, coarse, or scatological jokes for your buddies. Jokes about farting, belching, vomiting, and erectile dysfunction do not promote the kind of romantic ambience that you want to create. And if the girl you are flirting with is a blonde, hold the "dumb blonde" jokes—unless she invites you to do so by telling you one! As 2007 Pet of the Year Heather Vandeven put it, "Don't make fun of me, make fun of the situation." A little teasing, especially if she invites it by telling you a self-deprecating fact about herself, is fine; but don't make it harsh or mean-spirited. You want her to laugh with you, and she won't be laughing if you insult her or her values.

Add a Fleeting Touch

Once you engage her in a conversation, you can increase your connection by lightly, as if "accidentally," brushing your hand on her arm. Experiments have shown that a light, brief touch on the arm during a social encounter between strangers has both immediate and lasting positive effects. If she finds you likeable, a brief arm touch should prompt some reciprocal increase in intimacy, such as increased eye contact, more smiling, or more exchange of personal information. If you notice a positive response to your arm touch, wait a little while and then try a brief touch on her hand, which should prompt an even greater degree of intimacy. But keep those touches light and casual, and on her arm or hand only. There is no such thing as a "casual" touch on her breasts or ass; and if you grab for those areas before she is ready, you are likely to be grabbing your own penis when the night is over.

How to Nail the "Closing"

Good salespeople know when to close the deal—and so should you! Spend a little time getting to know her, then, when you feel that she has started to open up and share some personal information with you, this is the time to request her information and retreat. If you ask her out too soon, she will think you are only interested in her looks. While hot women like to be admired for their looks, they want to be appreciated for other qualities as well and considered more than a mere sex object. Make her feel special (intelligent, funny, interesting) by showing appreciation for her other qualities. Once she has shared some personal information about herself, you can act as if she has truly earned your interest. This way you will come across as a highly discriminating male, rather than a mere lustful "horn dog." And she will feel like a winner who has passed your "audition."

So once she reveals some personal data, it's time to excuse yourself (you are very busy!) and ask for her information. Unless she has given you a clear sign that she wants an invitation to your bedroom that very night, don't overstay your welcome by dragging out a conversation and telling her your whole life story. In fact, a lot of guys who make a positive first impression blow it by overextending this initial encounter. As one woman put it, "Some guys just seem to know what they are doing. They know how to approach you and just make you feel good. Then you get those nerds . . . who can't get anything right. They come on strong at first but can't keep it together . . . they just hang around until you dump them by going to the restroom or over to a friend to talk."[45]

So do not loiter around her. Instead, retain an aura of mystery; when you feel she is getting interested, tell her you have to run and ask her for her phone number or e-mail address. Make your inquiry direct and affirmative, such as "What is the best way to get in touch with you?" or "I am mostly available through e-mail. What is your e-mail address?" or "Do you have a cell phone, or should I call you at home?" Or tell her you enjoyed talking to her and you would love to meet again. Give her a piece of paper and a pen and tell her to write down her e-mail address, or pull out your cell phone and get ready to program in her number. Or give her your card and tell her, "Call me if you want to continue this conversation." If you really want to impress her, learn to memorize phone numbers and e-mail addresses using mnemonics.

If she seems obviously interested, you can turn the tables around and make it sound like she is the one asking for your number. You can say something to the effect of "Where can I find you so we can make arrangements to meet?" or "What steps would we have to take in order to make sure we meet again?" Or say, "I'll contact you tomorrow" or "I'd love to see that exhibit with you" or "Drop me an e-mail about that movie that you mentioned" and pretend to leave. Chances are she'll say, "But you don't have my number" or "You forgot to write down my number!" or "You never gave me your e-mail!" This way you are putting her in a position to ask for an exchange of information, making it sound like it was her idea in the first place.

Another option, especially effective if you feel that she is losing interest or playing aloof, is to say good-bye, start to leave, then turn around and say, "By the way, what's your e-mail address?" Try to sound friendly but casual and nonchalant as you say it—and by all means avoid begging her or trying to convince her to contact you. Remember: the image you want to project is that of a popular and busy guy who meets women all the time, and although you would enjoy hearing from her, you wouldn't be upset if you didn't. Once she agrees to share her e-mail address with you, give her a prepared paper and pen to write it down. For a bonus point, get yourself a fancy pen and some funny Post-its for writing notes. Women do notice all these little details and will use them to judge you. One guy at a club got a rise out of women by using a phallic-shaped pen with the inscription "Viagra" to write down his info. He was a pharmaceutical rep and got a ton of these pens for free—and they provided a great conversation starter and extender. While it is easier to get her e-mail address than her phone number, asking for a phone number will convey greater confidence on your behalf. Centerfold Courtney Taylor put it this way: "I would prefer the man to ask for my number. If a guy just asks for my e-mail address, then either a) he doesn't have the balls to ask for my number, or b) he isn't sure if he likes me right away. E-mail is OK for business, but not for romance. A guy should ask for both—that makes him seem confident." If you are feeling particularly ballsy, you can try to tease her into giving you her phone number by saying, "Write down your phone number too—unless you think I don't deserve it!" or "You can put down your phone number too, I promise not to sell it to telemarketers."

You can also prepare her for your phone call by telling her, jokingly, "When I call, I don't want you to act like I am some creditor calling. I want you to be excited about my call, OK?" You can then bring up this joke if she sounds grumpy when she picks up the phone.

If you want to know for sure if she is interested, you can skip exchanging information and just set up a date. Tell her that you will meet her at the same place or a local bar at a specific time that is convenient for both you and her in the next few days. If she agrees to that, chances are she will show up. Without a way to contact you directly, she will have no way of canceling the date other than calling the bar and leaving a message for you, upping her chances of either showing up or having to apologize and explain herself if she runs into you again. This approach works best if you live or work in close proximity to her and she knows that she has a high likelihood of running into you again.

Once you get her information, make sure to write down her name, date, and place you encountered her and any topics you might have discussed during your initial encounter. This is particularly important if you are out meeting a lot of women. If you are direct and confident and do not sound needy, lusty, or smitten by her, you will walk away not only with her number but with a combination to her heart as well!

TIP #12: To extend the conversation, use the following techniques:

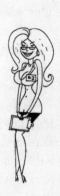

• Look for "word hooks" with which to continue the conversation

• Remember her name and use it often

• Listen more than speak

• Comment on what she says, and interpret how you think she feels

• Find common ground and stress similarity of your opinions

• Create a feeling of knowing each other for a while by using "we" statements

• Make nonoffensive jokes

• Touch her fleetingly on the arm

• Don't linger—get her info and exit pronto ✦

How to Approach a Group of Women

Approaching a group of women takes a bit more ingenuity than approaching a single woman does. If the women are standing together but their eyes are wandering everywhere, they are likely to be looking to pick up guys. If each one is taking turns to break away from the group and head over to the bathroom alone, they are definitely on the prowl and are there to pick up guys. However, if they are huddled together, giggling, and snickering as they check out guys, do not make your approach. Chances are they are out on a male-bashing night. When you do approach a group, do not go after a particular woman. Instead, throw out a question to them, or ask for their opinion or advice: "I need a feminine perspective. My buddy is getting married and I am at a loss as to what to get him." Women love it when men ask their opinions, and by approaching the entire group, rather than a particular woman, you will get them to compete with each other for your attention.

It's a guy's worst nightmare. You think she is ready to fall into your arms and say yes when you get around to asking for her number, but, instead, she cuts you dead. You desperately wish you could have interpreted her level of interest in you with more accuracy. Well, here are some nonverbal signs to watch for . . .

Top 10 Signs She Is Interested in You

1. Smiling or giggling at your jokes. When a woman is interested, she will smile coyly and laugh at your jokes, even bad ones. Wink at her, and see if she smiles. If she starts to laugh and act jovial in your presence, she is probably quite interested. When women are interested, they want to appear to be lots of fun. But make sure that her giggle is not a nervous habit, because the last thing you want is her snickering when you take your clothes off.

2. Smoothing or tossing her hair, or swirling it around her fingers. Hair play is a subtle invitation to foreplay. It's a suggestion as to what she would like you to do with your hands. But make sure she is not pulling her hair out—that could mean she is suffering from an impulse disorder called trichotillomania—unless you like your women bald.

3. Fidgeting, or fumbling an object, such as her glass. Signs of nervousness means her heart is going pitter-patter at the sight of you. Of course, it could also mean she is a klutz or strung out on some bad shit, so you have to assess this clue carefully.

4. Flushing or blushing when you look at her or pay her a compliment. Give her an intimate compliment, like "Wow, you have such succulent lips" and see if she blushes or if she calmly responds, "Yes, I just got my collagen injection." In the latter case, you might as well move on.

5. Pouting or puckering her mouth. Licking her lips, or a straw, or the edge of a glass she is holding is also a good sign. It means she's thinking of kissing or being kissed. It could also mean that she is dehydrated from doing too much Ecstasy, so don't be too literal in interpreting this sign.

6. Stuttering or stumbling over words. When women feel sexual attraction, their voices become higher in pitch, their speech patterns might change, and they might have trouble expressing themselves calmly. Of course, it could also mean she has a speech impediment, or an anxiety disorder, so don't take this as a sign of interest if this is the ONLY sign.

7. Moving or leaning toward you. This is an especially favorable sign. It means she is focused on you and feeling a desire for a higher degree of intimacy. When you observe this behavior, it is a good time to stoke up the heat of your conversation.

8. Fondling or stroking an object, such as her purse, or better yet, herself. If she is caressing her face or body, such as the back of her hands, the front of her thighs, or her breasts, turn on your penile radar. These are nearly infallible signs of her sexual interest. Unless there is a porn video playing, or a stripper dancing in the room, which could account for her arousal, you should be checking your condom supply.

9. Staring or gazing at you intently; then when you look at her, she lowers her eyes. This prolonged staring, called by anthropologists the "copulatory gaze," is a strong signal of her interest in you. Just make sure she is not staring at the guy behind you. Wandering eyes, on the other hand, is a sign she is looking for better prey.

10. Touching or brushing against your body. When a woman initiates physical contact, it is a clear indicator of her desire for physical intimacy. When she keeps on touching your arm or leg as you talk, or continually brushes up against you as you walk, it is time to pop the question "Your place or mine?"

Signs She Is Not Interested

+ She avoids eye contact

+ She doesn't smile or fakes a smile

+ She leans away from you

+ She answers in monosyllables

+ Her shoulders sag

+ She locks a "rescue me" look with someone else

+ She looks at her watch

+ She is tapping her foot

+ She is fidgeting

+ She is giving you a blank stare

Myth Rebuffed: HOT WOMEN GET
APPROACHED ALL THE TIME.

This is not true. Hot women get stared at, whistled at, and harassed by creeps more than average women do. But they are less likely to be approached by average men because men tend to be more intimidated by them.

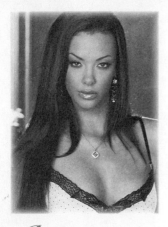

2005 *Pet* of the Year Runner-up Natalia Cruze prefers dark-skinned men and has dated, among others, a musician and a choreographer, as well as several atheletes.

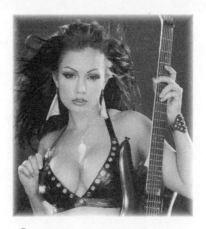

September 2000 Pet of the Month Aria Giovanni looks for a guy who is family-oriented and will be a good provider. She also likes a man to be "honest, intelligent, and affectionate."

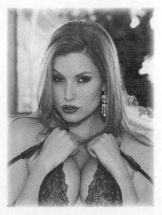

2006 *Pet* of the Year Jamie Lynn loves to date "a man who can get his hands dirty, rough on the edges."

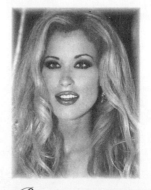

2004 *Pet* of the Year Runner-up Courtney Taylor has dated a few musicians, but prefers the men she dates to "have graduate degrees" and "to stimulate me both physically and intellectually."

PART 2

The Skill of Seduction:
Dating and Mating

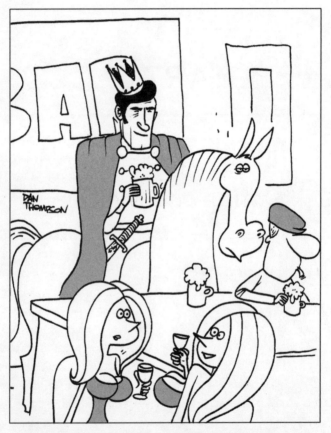

"I'm getting a vibe that the guy at the end of the bar
might be right for me."

Seduction is the desire of being overwhelmed, taken beyond.
— Daniel Sibony, *L'Amour Inconscient*

Hunt, pursue and capture are biologically programmed into the male sexuality. — Camille Paglia

Before we get into the logistics of a successful first date, let me give you a quick crash course on the way women think. Although women enjoy sex just as much men do—under the right circumstances—very few of them seek purely casual sexual encounters. Indeed, a majority of women yearn for *intimate* sex—which does not necessarily mean commitment but does imply emotional involvement beyond the mere biological act. Even the most liberated woman subconsciously prefers intimate sex to the totally casual variety, because for biological, evolutionary, and sociological reasons, the female brain is programmed to seek love, attachment, and bonding. From a biological perspective, after experiencing sexual pleasure, a woman's cerebral cortex secretes a far greater amount of the hormone oxytocin than a man's brain does. Oxytocin is known as the "attachment" or "bonding" hormone because it makes us want to cuddle after sex and is the primary driving force in our brains behind the desire for connection or intimacy. It is also exceedingly pleasurable in its effect on the mind. Because they experience such a strong oxytocin "rush" after sex, women generally are attracted to men who they believe can provide them with the kind of sexual intimacy that they subconsciously crave.

Moreover, years of evolution have shaped the female psyche to prefer sexual encounters that have at least the potential to turn into long-term romances. After all, prior to the invention of contraception, every time a woman engaged in a sex act she risked becoming pregnant—and subsequently saddled with the long-term responsibility of raising her offspring. And in peril-fraught prehistoric times, few women were able to rear an offspring on their own; for our ancient ancestors, single motherhood was hardly a viable option. Thus, centuries of evolution weeded out those promiscuous women who failed to secure a mate for breadwinning and protection of her young, and instead favored those who engaged in sexual acts selectively, such as by first assuring that their partners were genuinely interested in them. Given the millions of years that this evolutionary bias has been influencing women's minds, it is understandable that women prefer not to hop into bed with just any old Joe.

Of course, today's woman is no longer bound by the same restrictions that burdened her ancestors. She no longer depends on a man to protect her cave from predators or to hunt down a mammoth; and she can now earn her own living and decide whether she wants to get pregnant or not. But although the circumstances have changed, the female psyche is forever imprinted by our evolutionary past. And in many subtle, and some overt, ways, our society continues to propagate the notion that every woman needs romance and love in order to enjoy sex—and in order to feel truly fulfilled and alive.

For example, despite our postfeminist rhetoric about independent, self-actualized women not needing that old-fashioned storybook romance, little girls still grow up indoctrinated by fairy tales of beautiful princesses; almost every such tale seems to imply that a woman needs love in order to "live happily ever after." After all, both Snow White and Sleeping Beauty could only be awakened by a kiss from a prince who fell in love with them, rescuing them from their eternal slumber. The only way Cinderella escaped her gloomy, subservient fate was by capturing the heart of a prince. And it was Belle's falling in love with a hideous Beast that secured the happy ending of that fairy tale. These stories, and many other childhood fables, make little girls yearn to be such beauties them-selves and to have their Prince Charming come and sweep them off their feet—reinforcing their need for romance, love, and belonging, which was implanted in women by evolution and is supported by their biology.

And the prettier the girl, the more she identifies with the beauti-ful princesses in these stories. Indeed, the praise she gets for her looks convinces her that she too will have a fairy-tale romance. It is no wonder that deep inside the heart of every girl and the soul of every woman is the hope of falling in love with her very own knight in shining armor. So your challenge, in trying to score with the hottest women, is to create the possibility in her mind that you are her potential prince. This does not mean that you necessar-ily have to look like some movie Romeo. Remember, even in the fairy tales, women are willing to kiss (and screw) a lot of frogs in order to find their prince; and they have the ability to discover a real prince by his character, as in "Beauty and the Beast." But given the way a woman's mind works, you should never let a woman feel like all you are interested in is sex. Hot women are particularly per-ceptive on this score because they have been hit on, and even used, by men for sex much more often than average women.

Instead, the less eagerness to get her in bed that you show her, and the more she believes that you might be that knight in shining armor, the faster she will end up in your arms. Thus, everything you do from the minute you get her number should be oriented toward projecting that mysterious, nonchalant, gallant image of a potential knight—especially one who is willing to offer her that emotional connection her mind craves.

Eleven

Times and Places:
Planning Your First Contact

WHEN TO MAKE YOUR NEXT PITCH

As you walk out of Starbucks with a still-hot grande Raspberry Mocha Frappuccino in your hand and the piece of paper with her number, the number begins to burn a hole in your pants pocket. Whatever it takes, resist the temptation to dial her number "just to check" if she gave you the right one. Sadly, this has happened to me on a number of occasions—a guy would call me a few minutes after I gave him my number and then exclaim on the phone when I would pick up, "I just can't believe it's actually you!" Or worse yet, dial my number right in front of me to see if my phone would ring. Needless to say, I *never* returned their phone calls.

In the same vein, under no circumstances should you dial the number and hang up when she picks up. She will know it's you, and she will immediately downgrade you to her geek list. Instead, write her number down in your "black book" or daily planner and plan your strategy for the next few days. The first question you have to answer is, How long should you wait before contacting her? This is a hotly debated topic among dating experts, with some recommending a few days and others urging a wait of as long as a week. My advice—don't stress over it. As long as you don't bug her the same day, you will fare just fine in her eyes, whether you call her in a day or five days. The ideal time to wait is probably a couple of days, but remember, the longer you wait, the higher the likelihood that she will meet someone else, change her mind, or forget about you. Hot women are hot property, and their circumstances can change quite rapidly. They also know that men want them and might see through a contrived attempt to play cool. Some of them might also take offense if you wait too long to call them, or might get defensive and play harder to get as a result. For that reason, I do not recommend waiting more than four to five days to call her.

Here is my rough-and-ready calculation as to how the average hottie judges a man, based on his calling times:

TIME ELAPSED AFTER MEETING HER	HER THOUGHTS ABOUT YOU
A few minutes later	Control freak or, worse, a psycho
A few hours later	Needy loser
That same evening	Desperado with no life
The next morning	Eager beaver
In one or two days	Interested and following up
In four days	Busy or trying to play cool
After five days	Busy, disorganized, or too nervous to call earlier
More than a week	Busy, or two-timer, has a girlfriend or wife
Two weeks +	Player or jerk

Moreover, if she seemed obviously interested, I would call sooner rather than later because her interest was an indication that she does not have another guy in her life right now. How can you tell that she was interested? The eye contact she made during your initial conversation, the fact that she smiled a lot, asked you questions about yourself—all were clues, but they are not always reliable. After all, women are experts at feigning interest for the sole purpose of getting rid of a guy; and the hottest women have the most practice in doing just that. The best measure of her interest is the information (or lack thereof) she gives you to contact her. The more she gives, the more ready she is to receive your attention.

Here is a quick chart that rates the level of her interest on a 10 to 1 scale, with 1 being the highest interest:

SCALE OF HER INTEREST AS REFLECTED BY THE INFO EXCHANGE

(10) Took your number

(7.5) Wrote down her e-mail

(6.0) Gave you her e-mail + name

(4.5) Gave you her e-mail, phone number, + name

(2.5) Gave you her card + cell on back

(1) Gave you her card, cell, e-mail, + request for your info

For those who agonize over the "when should I call" issue, or who want some rule of thumb that takes the guesswork out of initiating that first call, just use the numbers above as the approximate call date for each situation; that is, the woman rating you a "1" on her interest scale should be called in 1 day, the woman rating you "2.5" should be called between two and three days following your first meeting, and so on.

When it comes to e-mail, you can contact her even sooner—as soon as the next day. I consider e-mails to be more convenient and far less intrusive than phone calls. A woman can ignore an e-mail for a few days if she doesn't feel like responding right away, while a phone call from you could put her on the spot or catch her when she is in a rush, in a bad mood, or on the other line. If she does not recognize you on the phone, she might feel like a fool or blow you off, while you can always include a flattering photo of yourself in the body of your e-mail to remind her of who you are, especially if your meeting was fleeting and it has been a few days since you met. (If you do enclose a photo, embody it in the text of your e-mail at the end of your message and make it look like it is part of your e-mail signature. Do not put it in the beginning with the words *Do you remember me?*)

Another advantage of e-mailing her is that it gives you time to compose a clever message without having to be quick on your feet and it won't betray any nervousness that you might still have about asking out hot women. Many guys are better writers than they are conversationalists; using e-mail helps them build a positive image in a woman's mind before going out on a date is even mentioned. Personally, I prefer scheduling all of my meetings via e-mail. I often check messages on my cellphone while driving or multitasking, and as a result I don't always have a pen handy—or I write the number down on some random piece of paper I cannot locate later. E-mails, on the other hand, are hard to "lose," and they are always there to remind her of your interest.

But e-mail does not create the same aura of intimacy as a personal phone call does, nor does it enable her to gauge your sincerity or the sound and timbre of your voice. While an e-mailed request to go out might be easily dismissed or ignored by a woman who is interested but wavering (or maybe considering dumping or two-timing her current boyfriend), a telephonic request is harder to turn down. So your best approach, even if you have exchanged a few e-mails, is to use the phone for making your first real pitch. However, just like a pitcher going over the hitters he is going to face in an upcoming game, you need to plan this first call carefully.

TIP #13: Contact her in two to four days after getting her information, depending on the degree of her interest. You can e-mail or text message her even sooner. If you have reached RIS, call her. Otherwise, use text messaging or e-mail to gauge her interest. ✦

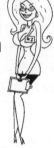

To Call or to E-mail—That Is the Question

E-MAIL OR TEXT MESSAGE HER A DATE IF

- You haven't gotten to RIS
- You met her briefly in a dark place
- Your voice tends to quiver
- She wasn't particularly interested

CALL HER TO SET UP A DATE IF

- She asked you to call her
- She wrote down her cellphone number
- You have a great voice
- You sound confident on the phone.

WHERE TO TAKE HER ON THE FIRST DATE

Before you make that first call or write that e-mail inviting her out, you need to plan where to take her. You need to be positive and have specific plans, rather than leave the decision up to her. Women like decisive, dominant men, and if you let her decide where to go, she is likely to perceive you as unimaginative and meek. Remember, you want to be her Prince Charming; princes do not ask others to decide things for them. So, have at least one specific date in mind when you call, and maybe a backup idea if she doesn't buy your first choice.

Of all the possible choices for a first date, I still believe—despite all the so-called dating gurus' contrary assertions—that a dinner date at a nice restaurant is the absolutely best place for that first serious get-together. I suspect that dating began when the first caveman brought a haunch of mammoth meat to the object of his desires and offered her a piece in return for a good screw. Well, things might have changed, but people haven't evolved that much since those early days. Women still respond positively to good food—indeed, the feeling of well-being that follows a satisfying meal often puts her in the mood for more intimacy. And offering her a tasty morsel from your plate, or "courtship feeding" as Helen Fisher puts it,[46] can be a step on the way to romance. Moreover, a restaurant is a perfect place for easy conversation, and that is a key element of any first date. As noted above, women not only like to talk; talking is one of their primary ways of evaluating potential love interests. So the combination of simultaneously nourishing her body and brain to begin building that intimacy which will lead to the bedroom makes a restaurant date the clear first choice.

Obviously, if you don't want to spend money on dinner, you can ask her to join you for lunch or a cup of coffee during her coffee break, but some women don't go out to lunch, and others tend to join their colleagues. In addition, if you work at the opposite side of town, lunch might not be a convenient option for either of you. Finally, she is more likely to be in a work mode during lunch or coffee break, and more likely to have her guard up. Thus, although lunch is not a bad date, a dinner date allows you more time to get to know, evaluate, and impress her.

I am not alone in this preference. Most of the models I interviewed for this book listed "dinner and drinks at a nice restaurant" as
their first choice for an initial date. Pet of the Year Julie Strain didn't
mince words: "Feed me or fuck off" was her comment on what a
guy should do to capture her interest. Indeed, a restaurant date was
favored as either the first or second choice by every hot model who
answered my questionnaire, so you can't go wrong with offering to
take her to dinner on that critical first date.

▶ *Most hot women prefer having dinner on the first date.*

Now where to invite her to dinner? Some women like to be given
the choice. If you don't know her preferences or tastes, it is not
a bad idea to have a few possible suggestions in mind and then
let her pick. If she has a favorite restaurant and offers it as an
alternative to what you suggested, you might want to go with her
choice; but otherwise, you want to appear decisive and knowledge-
able about restaurants in the area. The phone call you are planning
might go something like this:

> YOU: So how about dinner this Thursday?
> SHE: OK, that sounds nice.
> YOU: If you like Italian, I know this great bistro in Little
> Italy—you know, the kind where the food is really great,
> while the atmosphere is really rustic. Or if you prefer Asian
> food, I know this fantastic dim sum place where they serve
> you like 200 varieties of dishes and it's all-you-can-eat. Or if
> you have another favorite. . . . ? (Pause to let her name it.)
> SHE: Oh, I love Asian food. Let's go there.

By naming the choices for her, you show that you are an "in
charge" kind of guy; by allowing her to suggest another alternative, you show her that you respect her tastes and desires too. You
don't want to give her an open-ended "Where do you want to go?"

option. This is especially dangerous if you are trying to stay on a
dating budget—high-maintenance beauties are likely to name a
gastronomic feast in one of the top Zagat restaurants. And you
want to make sure that you do not bring all of your dates to the
same place, lest some uncouth waiter were to comment on how
nice it is to be seeing you every week with a different beauty. If
in your initial meeting you learned she liked a particular food, or
was of a particular ethnic background, you will want to choose
a place that will appeal to her tastes. Try scouting out the best
places in advance, even before making that first call, but if you
don't have a clue as to her favorite foods, choose restaurants that
you like and are familiar with. This gives you the added advantage of knowing what dishes to recommend to her, or of impressing her by being greeted as a returning or frequent diner by the
maitre d'.

▸ *Choose the restaurant consistent with your prototype, as she will
associate the ambience with you.*

The ambience of the place you choose is almost as important as
the food, as she will subconsciously associate the place with you,
transferring the emotions she feels there to you.[47] So if you are trying to project the prototype of a modern, progressive male, choose
a restaurant with a contemporary theme. If she is into antiques
and seems to have a penchant for old-fashioned gentlemen, choose
a place with a more Victorian look. I was really impressed when
a guy who met me at a Halloween party where I was dressed up
in an Alice in Wonderland outfit invited me to a small and little
known but undeniably charming Manhattan restaurant named
Alice's Tea Cup. By naming a restaurant that matches what you
know of her tastes, it shows her you paid attention during your initial conversation. That always gets her attention!

However, even if you want her to view you as a highly accomplished guy with the means to support her, do not choose the most

expensive restaurant around.[48] Subconsciously, she could end up thinking, *The main reason why I had fun on that date is because he took me to that ritzy restaurant everyone is talking about.* You want her to think that the main reason she had fun was because you were such an interesting guy. Besides, beautiful women are constantly being propositioned by rich creeps; and, in their minds, high-price restaurants may be associated with such "indecent proposals." Another reason not to choose a very posh place, even if you are swimming in money, is the establishment of unreasonable expectations. Once you set the bar at a high stake, it will be impossible to lower it without disappointing her. She will expect you to entertain her in the same expensive style for the length of your dating, and unless you are willing to do that, start at a level you can afford without going broke. Save the ritzy places for later in the relationship when you want to give her a special treat.

▶ *Choose a romantic restaurant that is not too expensive and that will make her feel strong, positive emotions.*

Similarly, choose locations that will make her feel strong, positive emotions. Research has shown that there is a strong link between emotional arousal and sexual attraction. One way to stir up her emotions is to take her to a place that will make her reminisce about her childhood or that will have a personal, intimate association for her. If she grew up in New Orleans, invite her to a Cajun restaurant; if she majored in biology, suggest checking out the Museum of Natural History. For example, being of Russian descent, I prefer Russian food, and any guy who invites me to a Russian restaurant will score major points in my book. While an invitation to Samovar, an expensive Manhattan restaurant, would impress me, one to a small, less pricey but far more charming one such as Uncle Vanya would score higher points. And being brave enough to meet me for dinner at one of the authentic places in Brighton Beach's Little Russia, followed by a concert by my favorite native singer, would probably guarantee at least a passionate makeout session afterwards. Why? Because it would demonstrate a willingness to be immersed in my culture without the xenophobia so many foreign beauties are faced with, and it would make me feel an immediate sense of kinship with you. So if you are planning to go out with foreign-born hotties, make sure to make your date a culturally sensitive one by researching her country of origin in advance. If you can make her feel nostalgic melancholy in your presence, she may be soon reminiscing about her childhood in your postcoital embrace!

A dinner date by itself is an OK starter date, but if you can combine it with another activity, it gives you more time to get to know each other and provides more opportunities for fun—which will leave her with a positive opinion of you, no matter how smooth you are as a conversationalist. The most popular activities among my Penthouse friends are—believe it or not—cultural events like art galleries, concerts, or stage shows, or physical activities like bowling, ice skating, horseback riding, or walks in the park. Nature-oriented settings, like botanical gardens, a park, or even the beach, offer a little mixture of both. If you choose a cultural activity, try to make it an "arousing" one, like an exhibit of modern (or ancient) erotic art, or a moving concert or stage play. Physical activities should get the adrenaline flowing but not be so competitive as to turn her off. Such activities give you something interesting to talk about over dinner, so make sure you time the activity to fit your restaurant reservation.

Movies, although popular with a lot of daters, are actually a bad choice for a first date! Most of the hot models who answered my questionnaires listed movies near the bottom of the list of choices, just above strip clubs as the worst choice for a first date. Movies are disfavored because you can't talk during them, or look in her eyes; and you don't know each other well enough to expect a good cuddle—which is the primary plus for a movie date. So other than the entertainment value of the film, there is little in a movie to advance the relationship. If you do choose a movie with dinner, try to pick a chick flick or something you know she likes. My friend and fellow Pet Courtney Taylor is passionate about Woody Allen movies, so you will score points with her by taking her to one of his classics. If you know me, you know I am into foreign films, particularly French dramas, so you would impress me by taking me to one. But you don't usually know enough about the woman to make such an informed choice on the first date, so save the movies for when you have her hooked—and when you can use the dark theater to get in some exciting "public" sex or at least a hot makeout.

▸ *Choosing exciting places for your first date increases the chances of her falling for you.*

One possible choice for a good first date is an activity with a touch of danger or frightfulness. Amusement parks, hot air balloon rides, paintball games, rock climbing machines, kayaking, parasailing, sky gliding, or even some fast horseback riding are potentials here. There is a definite psychological link between danger and physical/romantic attraction.[49/50] A little anxiety leads us to eroticize the situation and imbue a potential partner with an added romantic appeal because our brains respond to the surge of adrenaline in our bodies by attributing situational anxiety to interpersonal attraction. So if you happen to be a daredevil and so is your quarry, by all means take her on an activity that will take her breath away. However, be sure that both you and she—ask her first—are not afraid of heights or susceptible to motion sickness, as nothing ruins a date more than a bad case of puking. If she is not up for a physically arousing experience, you should try to choose an emotionally provoking one, such as a moving theatrical play, or a concert with a stimulating band or artist, or some emotionally charged art exhibit.

Unless she is a big sports fanatic, and it is her favorite team playing, I would not recommend taking a hottie to a sporting event. Taking her somewhere she'd be checking out all those highly masculine players might not bode well for you—particularly if you don't have a great physique.

People tend to make subconscious comparisons between their prospective partners and other prospects available. Studies have shown that men tend to judge their girlfriends as less attractive after checking out Playboy centerfolds. Although there is no comparable study on women, I suspect women are prone to the same subconscious comparisons, albeit to a lesser extent. I know from personal experience. Once I was invited to a basketball game by a weatherman, who had a very cute face and was popular with women in Philly inspite of his somewhat short stature and unimpressive physique—TV made him look bigger than he was. We sat in the very front row, normally assigned to media guests only. I am not a big sports fan and was bored stiff, until the basketball hit me right on the head—to my utmost embarrassment! The player, who came to apologize to me after the game, ended up slipping me his number. Next to this tall athlete, the weatherman looked particularly diminutive and emmasculated. Needless to say—instead of hooking up with the weatherman, I ended up going out with the athlete!

There are some semipopular dating places that you absolutely need to discard as far as a first date is concerned. Strip clubs, nightclubs, and parties with your friends are definitely out. You don't want to be caught checking out another woman while just getting to know a new hot honey; conversations are about impossible in loud clubs; and your odds of having her spot some other Prince Charming are greater in such places. Parties with your friends might sound like a good idea, but as Playmate Charlotte Kemp put it, "I felt like I was on display and being judged . . . and you can be sure I never went out with him again!" The only thing worse is taking her to your parents' house or to some family gathering. That would get you demoted to "loser" status by just about every Playmate or Pet I know. Here is a list of some other "Hall of Shame" first dates:

Worst Places to Take Her on a First Date

1. Fast-food restaurant. No matter how broke or starved you are, do not take her to a place that even remotely resembles a fast-food joint or a truck-stop diner. No matter how proletarian her views are, fast food will get you a fast boot!

2. Funerals or cemeteries. Unless she loves vampires or she is goth, avoid anything related to death and dying. I don't know any hot women who list "grave rubbings" as their hobby.

3. Your kids' school play or birthday party. No matter how adorable your kids seem to you, chances are she will find them to be an annoying reminder that some other woman claimed your affection first. To avoid losing points early in the game, keep your rugrats under the rug until she gets into the "love me, love my dog" stage of romance.

4. Your parents' house. There are innumerable reasons to avoid introducing your date to your parents for as long as possible. Chances are you resemble your father—and she will get a mental picture of what you will look like in thirty years, with a potbelly and hairy ears. And your mother might slip and remind you to wash your hands before dinner again.

5. Strip club, X-rated films, or swingers parties. Rule of thumb: avoid any place that has scantily clad women, explicit depiction of sexual activities, or sexually aggressive males on the first date. The only exception is The Museum of Sex or an erotic art exhibit, particularly if she displays an intellectual curiosity about it or claims to be a sexpert, like *moi*.

6. Party with your ex. Even if you parted on the best of terms with your ex, avoid having her in close proximity to your date for as long as possible. Women hate being replaced and will go to great lengths to prevent their ex from getting laid again.

7. Church (baptism, wedding, etc). I believe that religion is the absolute antithesis of sex, as it seems to exist to remind us that we are going to pay dearly for everything fun that we do in this life.

8. Window shopping. When it comes to hot women, there is no such thing as window shopping. Remember when the Red Queen introduced Alice to her food? She said, "Alice, meet the pudding, pudding meet Alice!" then told Alice now that they were acquainted, Alice was not to eat the pudding. Well, don't make the same mistake with your date. She doesn't want to "meet the clothes," she wants to wear them!

TIP #14: Choose several date ideas and offer them to her. Do not let her offer suggestions unless you are ready to pay top dollar for her culinary quest. Choose places that are consistent with your prototype, as she will transfer the ambient feelings about the place onto you. Take her to places that would make her feel strong positive emotions, like a concert, a venue that would evoke nostalgia, a restaurant from her homeland, or an activity that would give her butterflies in her stomach, like a hot-air balloon, or roller-coaster ride, or a tear-jerking show (or movie if there is one she really wants to see). ✦

Twelve

First Call and Confirmation: Asking Her Out

You know what charm is: a way of getting the answer yes without having asked any clear question.   —ALBERT CAMUS

THAT NERVE-WRACKING FIRST CALL

Now that you have set the time to call her and planned the first date you want to take her on, it is time to make that call. For many guys, especially those who have not achieved full RIS (Rejection Immunity State), this is "nervous time." So before you make the call, you might want to review chapter 5 and harden your heart against any fear of being turned down. You want to be the self-confident superhero you think you are, and no mere woman, however beautiful and sexy, can stop you from being the man you believe yourself to be.

Moreover, before you pick up the phone and impulsively dial her number, make sure you recall her name, any nickname or family name she has disclosed to you, any topics you might have discussed with her, and any specifics about her hair, face, and body you noticed about her. If you are out and about meeting a lot of women—as you should!—it's easy to get confused, especially if you failed to follow my advice to write down her information right away next to her number. The last thing she wants to hear as she answers her phone is "Hi, um, I don't remember your name, but we met last week . . ." Other than mentioning her by name and remembering the specifics of your meeting, the content of the follow-up lines is not as crucial as their tone. As with your opening lines, the key is to sound nonchalant, composed, and not too eager, but not altogether disinterested. Remind yourself that you have been invited to call—giving you her number was a clear indication that she will welcome hearing from you.

▸ *Go over your confidence-building strategies before dialing her number.*

The mental attitude of being "an invitee" versus "a trespasser" or a nuisance will reflect in your voice. It is a good idea to practice, in your mind at least, that first call, until you can deliver your dating proposal with the right degree of confidence and nonchalance. Don't be embarrassed by rehearsing this call. A friend of mine who is a famous trial lawyer says he rehearses in his mind, sometimes for hours, every key argument, cross-examination, or direct examination—even after thirty years' experience in the courtroom! So rehearsing is a good thing when it comes to making a good impression on those you want to impress. Practice asking for her, making sure you pronounce her name correctly, and do a mental rundown of what you would like to say. Know your availability in advance so that you can offer her an alternative date if she happens to be unavailable on the first day you propose. And for God's sake, do not call her when you are drunk—or even slightly inebriated! If she picks up on your slurred speech, she will assume that you needed to get drunk to muster the courage to call her.

Another important decision is what time of day to call her. I absolutely detest when I get phone calls too early in the morning before I get a chance to get my bearings together. Many hot women are not early birds—some are out partying late at night, and most are busy beautifying themselves in the morning. Your best bet is to avoid calling her before 10 a.m. or after 10 p.m., with the best times depending on whether she gives you her home, cellular, or work number. Because very few hot women give out their home numbers, and most do not like to be bothered at work, your best bet is to call her cell phone. Evening hours are always better for connecting with her, as she is more likely to be in the mood for hooking up in the evenings.

TYPE OF NUMBER	BEST TIME TO CALL
Cell phone	Between 5 and 9 p.m.
Home	Between 6 and 9 p.m.
Work	Between 10 and 11 a.m., before it gets hectic or she goes to lunch

Do not call in the morning unless she specifically asked you to.

OK, it's now the hour and day, and you are practiced and have a date planned. Go ahead and dial that number you won from her on your first meeting.

When she picks up, identify yourself and mention the place where you met. You can then ask her how she has been doing or ask her about her day. If she mentioned a specific hobby or interest during your initial meeting, you can weave it into your dialogue. Be concise and to the point, do not drag out the conversation, and, to the extent possible, be the first to terminate the call and say good-bye. Here's a sample:

SHE: Hello?

YOU: Nanette? It's Rob, we met at Starbucks last week. You promised you'd be excited when I called.

SHE: Oh, yeah, what's up?

YOU: I am on the way to a gym. How are you, Nanette?

SHE: I am fine, getting ready to have dinner.

YOU: You mentioned you were born in France, so you probably like French cuisine.

SHE: I sure do.

YOU: There is a new French restaurant that just opened not far from me. I plan to check it out next week, do you want to join me?

SHE: OK, why not?

YOU: How about next Thursday, March third, at 6 p.m.

SHE: I can't make it till about 7.

YOU: OK, 7 p.m. Let's meet at Starbucks and go from there.

SHE: OK.

YOU : Well, gotta go. Enjoy your dinner. See you next Thursday!

To many guys, the example above will seem overly brief and unfriendly. However, with a woman, it is always important to maintain an air of mystery. You don't want to drone on in that first call. Instead, you want to have her thinking about you, wondering about you, and looking forward to your date. Remember, she hasn't rehearsed this call, or likely even thought a lot about what you or she might say if you did call. She might have been hoping you would call, but she won't have a date all planned; you were the one taking charge when you made the call, so you should be the one to ring off. Besides, while you might be able to read her desire to hear from you in her voice, you will not be able to judge her reactions to any substantive conversation over the phone. You need the nonverbal clues of face-to-face conversation to get a good idea of the impression you are making. So keep it short, and hold the "big stuff" for your date.

Whenever you can, suggest meeting in the middle of the week as opposed to a weekend. As you will see later, you need to act like a very busy guy with a full social schedule, and suggesting a weekend date works against that concept. You don't want to come across as a guy whose weekends are free! She is also more likely to be available during the week, minimizing your chances of being turned down. If she has nothing planned for Wednesday night, why not go on a dinner date with an interesting guy? Finally, restaurants and all the other venues you plan on taking her to are less likely to be crowded during the week, giving you more privacy to engage in deep conversation.

▶ *Invite her out in the middle of the week, as opposed to a weekend, to show that you have a busy social schedule.*

If she sounds rushed or frazzled when she picks up, do not drag out the conversation. You can give her your phone number and casually ask her to call you back when she has more time to talk. However, a better option is to ask her when she is available to chat and to tell her that you will contact her again at that time— this way you are making sure that she will not lose your information or forget to call you back. Do not lose your confidence if she sounds rushed or inattentive—women are much more likely to multiask than men, and she might be in the middle of driving, getting ready to go out, or in the company of family and friends. Do not take personally her inability to converse with you at that very moment. If you catch yourself making an internal negative attribution of the sort, like "If she really liked me she would have made the time to talk to me," immediately refute that thought by externalizing the situation: "She must be in the middle of something." Then make sure to follow up when you said you would; perseverance and reliability are impressive to a woman. Not calling her at the agreed-upon time in order to demonstrate that you are not smitten by her will not score you any points with her at this time—you are not in a position to play hard to get until you get her attention.

SHE: Hello.

YOU: Is this Victoria?

SHE: Yup, but I can't really talk right now.

YOU: No problem, when is a good time to call back?

SHE: Between 6 and 8 p.m.

YOU: I will talk to you then. Take care.

SHE: Bye.

If she is unavailable and someone else answers, do not hang up! Many guys immediately assume when they hear a male voice on the other line that it must be her boyfriend. In fact, it could be any male in her life—her father, her brother, her cousin, friend, or roommate, or merely someone who happens to pick up her phone, or even a wrong number! One time I ran into a guy who failed to contact me after I gave him my number. It turns out that he had indeed, called me, but he'd failed to leave a message after my nephew had mischievously answered my cell phone. The guy had assumed I was either married or had a son and had decided not to leave his information. Do not make any assumptions! If someone else answers her phone, simply ask for her, and if she is not available, leave your name and phone number. But don't give out any other information, even if the person answering tries to pry—you don't know her situation, and you don't want to cause any friction.

VOICE: Hello.

YOU: Hi, is Lexie there?

VOICE: No. Who is this?

YOU: This is John, I'd like to leave a message for her.

VOICE: Are you her personal trainer?

YOU: No.

VOICE. Oh. Some guy she met at the club?

YOU: I'd like to leave her a message, please. I am John Right, and my number is 555-1212. Just have her return my call.

VOICE: OK. I'll give her the message.
YOU: Thanks, and have a good day.

What if you leave her a message and she does not call back? I believe you should try to call her at least one more time, in case she accidentally erased your message, misplaced your number, or your message did not come through clearly on her cell phone's answering service. However, I would quit calling her after the second unreturned message. If you continue, you risk coming across as a stalker.

But what if you do reach her and she tells you that she cannot meet you because she is "busy"? How do you know whether this excuse is legitimate or just a thinly disguised attempt to blow you off? Women do use "I am so busy these days" and "It's been really crazy at work" as an excuse. To check if it is true, ask her to meet for a celebratory drink when her workload lightens up or when her project is done. If she gives you a specific deadline for her work, she is more likely to be telling the truth; if she is being evasive and perpetually busy, chances are she is using it as a polite excuse. You can increase your chances of overcoming her reluctance if you introduce an element of intrigue. Tell her you've got a special surprise for her that she would really like, or that you picked something up for her (never spend more than a few bucks on an initial gift, though). You can also tell her that you thought of a perfect nickname for her, or that you found out something important about her from your psychic friend—but you are only willing to share it with her tête-à-tête.

▸ *If she tells you that she is busy, lure her out by telling her you've got a surprise for her.*

Once you get her on the phone and your conversation is moving along, make sure to nail all of the details of the date, such as the exact time and location, and to reconfirm them at the end of the conversation if you end up chatting for a while (although you should try to hang up as soon as possible). A confirmation call the day before the date is also a good idea to prevent a no-show, particularly if she has a busy social calendar or seems flaky, or if you are setting up a date a week or more in advance. To make sure you have a reason to reconfirm closer to your date, leave some details of the date out of your initial phone call. For example, you can tell her that you will call her back later with the landmark of the location, cross street, or dress code. Don't just call to remind her of your date—it will sound obsessive and controlling.

DATE DETAILS TO SET UP IN THE FIRST PHONE CALL:

✦ What you are going to do

✦ When you will meet (date, day of the week, and hour)

✦ Where you will meet (name of the place and address)

DATE DETAILS TO SET UP IN THE CONFIRMATION PHONE CALL:

✦ Additional activities or details

✦ What the exact location is (landmark, cross street)

✦ The fact that you got the tickets or made reservations

✦ What the dress code is

✦ Who will drive, if necessary

Another way to contact her if you have her phone number is by text messaging her. It is less intrusive than a phone call and allows you to communicate with her in real time. If you have not reached the RIS state, you can use text messaging to test the waters.

If she gives you her e-mail address instead of her number, you can ask her out on a date without phone communication, but only after touching base with her first. The biggest disadvantage of communicating via e-mail is that you cannot hear how she reacts to your phone call. But it might serve to your advantage if you tend to get nervous or overly vigilant for any signs of rejection. In your initial e-mail, just say hello and bring up where you met. Keep the e-mail short and the tone light, but push for some level of feedback. Being able to grab her interest is always better than a boring e-mail like: "Hi, it's me John, we met the other night. How are you?" Instead, try something like this.

> Hi, Jaime. It's John, we met the other day at Starbucks. You mentioned you like foreign films. There is an awesome new French film that I have just seen. E-mail me and I'll tell you more about it.

After she responds, tell her you are considering seeing that movie again and ask her if she wants to join you. Although going to a movie theater is a less-than-ideal date, in this case demonstrating that you have the same interest in movies would score you a point or two. I know that a good steamy French movie or a Spanish film by Almodóvar would definitely tempt me to go out on a date.

If you have an instant message service, you can ask her if she has one. An instant messenger is a great way to keep communication flowing without worrying about how you sound. As much as many guys detest America Online for being overly pushy with their commercials, many hot women have AOL accounts and agree to chat on AOL instant messenger.

I Screwed Up by . . . Sounding Nervous

If you realize that you are sounding hesitant or out of breath, you can always blame it on the circumstances. If you feel her noticing the fact that you're pausing too long to collect your thoughts, say something like "Sorry, I am driving right now and I am a bit disoriented." If you sound out of breath or your voice falters, you can blame it on just having finished a workout: "I just got off the treadmill." Remember, she cannot see you, and your anxiety always seems worse to you than it is perceived by others.

Should I:

• Offer to pick her up? You might, although it is not necessary unless she mentions transportation problems. Never insist on it— it sounds too intrusive.

• Bring flowers? No. It looks too ingratiating and she will have to drag them around all night or leave them in her car and let them wither.

• Bring a gift? Generally, no, unless it is something inexpensive and has to do with her interests, such as a book or a collectible (for me, it's water globes).

TIP #15: Contact her between 10 a.m. and 10 p.m., introduce yourself, and set up the meeting. If she is unavailable and her voice mail picks up or someone else answers, do not hang up. Leave a very brief message and your phone number. If she doesn't call you back after two messages, forget about her. If you get her on the phone, set up the date after a brief talk, but leave out some unimportant details so that you have a reason to reconfirm the meeting; that way, you avoid her flaking out. ✦

Thirteen

Core Beliefs and Commonalities: Conversing on the First Date

I was on a date. I was really uncomfortable. My guts were churning—it was really awkward. So finally, I figured, hey, I'll just ask her, "What's your name?"   —GARY SHANDLING

Words have a place, but too much talk will generally break the spell, heightening surface differences and weighing things down. People who talk a lot most often talk about themselves. They have never acquired that inner voice that wonders, Am I boring you?"   —ROBERT GREENE, *The Art of Seduction*

The first date is always critical in scoring with a hot chick, as it will not only determine whether you will get more dates with her but will also set the level of her interest and desire for you. You might not get laid on that first date—and you shouldn't expect to in this day of AIDS-conscious women and with super- sexy women who have been propositioned for casual sex more times than you have had dates—but your chances of getting laid on later dates might well be determined by how well you pull off the initial dating experience with her. What you want to accomplish, regardless of how badly you would like to get into her pants immediately, is to have her see you as a possible romantic interest, a man she wants to spend more time with, and someone she would consider as a bedmate "when the time is right." This is how you go about it.

How to Go About Conversing on the First Date

Maintain Your Mystique

What you talk about on the first date is much more important than what you said when you first met her. At the initial meeting she was paying far more attention to your overall appearance and demeanor than to the content of your words. This time she will be heeding the message behind your words, figuring out if you are worth wasting her precious time on. If you kept your initial conversation short and finished it first, and did the same in your call to set up the date, she was probably left wondering what you are really like. Maintaining this mystique is one of the most important things you need to accomplish on the initial date—and for a while thereafter. Most guys get nervous around hot women and end up either clamming up or talking too much as a way of dealing with their anxiety. By doing the latter, they usually reveal too much of themselves, in effect "demystifying" their persona, which in turn prevents a very important psychological process from taking place.

When we first meet a person we like, we subconsciously engage in a psychological process of projective idealization, whereby we imbue the person with the qualities we find desirable in a mate. Do not be frightened by the complexity of the term—all it means is that we tend to imagine that that person fits our desired prototype, the "love map" we talked about earlier. In this process, we idealize the desired one and imbue him or her with the qualities we want them to have. However, if you reveal too much personal information too soon, she might soon realize that there is a discrepancy between her idealized you and the real deal. As her fantasy dissipates like the morning fog, she will feel disillusioned, and your chances of bedding her will dissipate as well!

For example, she might envision you as an independent guy who is "fully differentiated" from his family. If you reveal to her that every Sunday you have dinner at your mother's house, she might immediately dismiss you as a "momma's boy," just like her ex, whom she despised for catering too much to his parents. Of course, if you end up going out with her often, you will eventually reveal that info to her, but not until she has developed some attachment to you. Once a woman falls for a man, she is willing to overlook a lot of his negative traits (often in the hope that eventually he will change for her). On the first few dates, you want to keep those potential negative traits under wraps!

Be an Attentive Listener to Get Her to Open Up

Thus, your first-date conversational strategy should be to reveal as little about your inner world as possible and to learn as much as you can about her. This serves three purposes: (1) to maintain your mystique so that she can continue to project her idealized male image onto you; (2) to make getting into your inner world a challenge for her; and (3) to get to know her better so that you can then highlight your similarities and complementary differences as described below. Obviously, you shouldn't be evasive if she asks you a direct question, but you should not volunteer too much personal information or drone on about your life history. Use personal disclosure to highlight similarity with her viewpoints *after* she reveals her interests and convictions.

Here are some examples of the things you can feel confident in talking about on the first date ("hits") and some of the things you should not address ("misses"):

HITS	MISSES
Talking about her life, goals, job	Talking about her looks, sexual experience
Discussing celebrities' decisions	Admiring celebrities' money or looks
Discussing your ambitions, travel plans	Discussing your childhood, family, finances
Telling her about books you read	Telling her about computer games you play
Sharing shows you watch	Sharing sports statistics
Commenting on the ambience, service	Criticizing ambience, food, service
Sharing your hobbies	Droning on about your stamp collection
Mentioning your pet	Raving about your devotion to your pet
Discussing her past relationships	Criticizing your ex-girlfriends

Mostly, though, you want to encourage her to talk about herself. For most women, that is never a problem, as women love to talk far more than men do.[51] Women also feel good, physically, when they talk.[52] So it is easy to hold a conversation with a woman—just open a topic, be an active listener, and let her go! To encourage her to continue talking, employ a lot of empathizers, such as "I see what you mean," "Yes, you were right," "I can relate to that," and "I understand."

Delve Deeper in Her Mind

As noted above, the best topic for a first-date conversation is HER. Talking about her not only makes her feel good but it also allows you to gather information about her (which you will then use to highlight your similarities—a key element of bonding with her). Ask her about her occupation, her hobbies and interests, her aspirations and dreams, and act like you are really interested in what she has to say. The key, though, is to get her to talk about her *feelings,* as opposed to merely revealing factual information about herself. Women are emotionally oriented, so for them, being asked about their feelings is perfectly natural. This is exactly what mental health therapists do—they help us explore our emotions—and that is the reason why talk therapy makes us feel good.

As described earlier in chapter 10, try to use active listening techniques to paraphrase what she is saying. Reflect the feeling she is conveying by using phrases like "It must have been a really tough decision to give up your acting aspirations and leave L.A." Whenever she is describing a challenge she has overcome, use the "How did it make you feel?" question to show your interest in her emotions. Having said that, avoid clichéd questions she has been asked a million times, such as "How does it feel being so beautiful?" or "How did it feel posing nude?" By engaging in active listening and reflecting her emotions, you will be able to create instant rapport and transference, a process of redirecting upon you memories of positive past interactions.

Whereas you should bring up only positive information about your family (such as your dad's adoration for your mom) and keep totally mum about your prior relationships (unless you dated Ivanka Trump, then dumped her because you could not stand her dad), do inquire about her family and her prior relationships. If she tells you that she is close to her family, tell her you respect her for that because it shows that she is a caring human being (whether you believe it or not). For example, my sister takes care of our dad, who doesn't speak much English and can be quite demanding. She would only date men who expressed admiration for her caretaking abilities. If she brings up her prior relationships, inquire further about them. What did she like about her ex-boyfriend? Once she tells you, make a mental note to display that quality if you can. What was the reason they broke up? Whatever the reason, take her side (even if you totally disagree). Oh, he was a sports fanatic and never took her shopping on Sundays. You say, "Yeah, it's too bad some guys are so one-dimensional—you deserve a guy who is more into you than into some pro sports team."

Fish for Commonalities

As I mentioned in the first chapter, we are drawn to partners with similar attitudes, values, and interests. Research has consistently shown that attraction to a stranger is correlated with the degree of similarity that the subjects perceive.[53] Discovering that you have a similar outlook on life with someone gives you that feeling of déjà vu, the feeling that you have known each other for a long time, i.e., that "soul mate" feeling for which every woman yearns. Knowing that she has a lot in common with you is important to her because subconsciously she is evaluating your suitability as a long-term partner, and she instinctively knows that partners with similar attitudes have a much better chance of staying together after the initial passion cools off. Whether your views are actually consistent with hers or not is not that important at this point, both because a woman will frequently accommodate her views to a man's if she falls in love with him and because most guys are willing to alter their outlook on life quite a bit to accommodate the views of a sexy woman! But before you can make her feel like she has been searching for you all her life, you need to find out what her beliefs actually are (without being too obvious about it).

One of my friends was deeply infatuated with one of the Penthouse Pets. At one of the magazine's social gatherings, he began to put down and berate people who use drugs, thinking he would impress her with his clean-cut image. However, she took his comments as a personal offense, as she likes to smoke marijuana and was named the Ganja Queen of the Year for *High Times* magazine. As a matter of fact, a majority of hot models are prone to indulge in the use of illegal substances, so if you are morally opposed to such things, keep those views to yourself until you know whether your target is a user or an abstainer. Indeed, do not express any strong opinions until you get to know hers.

However, you don't have to be a yes-man, agreeing with everything she says. In fact, some verbal sparring about tangential issues can be used to incite her passion. However, agreeing with her on the major points, her core beliefs, will earn you major points. Studies show that it is not the number of similarities that brings people together but the intensity of their similarities regarding their major beliefs. For example, if she is an ardent animal-rights activist, merely joking that PETA stands for "people eating tasty animals" will probably lead to your getting a slap on the face (while mentioning that you volunteer at animal shelters will earn you at least a kiss, maybe more). Your agreement doesn't always have to be verbal, either. In fact, nonverbal behavior can speak volumes about your convictions. Watch for her reactions to the world around you and express the same emotions, but with even greater intensity. If she gives a bum a quarter as you are walking down the street, outdo her and give him a dollar.

As I mentioned above, all women will subconsciously evaluate you as a long-term partner, even if they THINK they just want to have a one-night stand. As Rita Rudner put it, "When I meet a man, I look at him and ask, 'Is this the man I want my children to spend every other weekend with?'" For that reason, mentioning facts and opinions that would make you a desirable husband and father will always give you points—even if she is already married with kids and is only looking for an extramarital swing. One time I met this guy who was not really my type, but what ultimately made me go out with him was the fact that he said, "I am looking for a woman to worship. My father to this day worships my mother and brings her breakfast in bed." That kind of worship I just had to experience, at least once!

Elicit Her Core Beliefs

Ultimately, what you want to do is find out the values, or core beliefs, that comprise her worldview, from which she derives her views on life, pursuit of happiness, and relationship expectations. Once you tap into her core beliefs, you can express agreement with them, making her feel like you are her long-lost soul mate. Here are the questions you ultimately want to obtain answers to:

• What does she seek in life?

• What does she wish she could have?

• What does she think she deserves?

• What did she once have but lost?

• What is she afraid of?

• What makes her happy?

• What turns her on?

However, most of the time you cannot ask these questions directly. Instead, you need to work them into general questions about her life. For example, you can ask her about what her childhood was like, what she likes about her current job or the town she lives in, or where she would like to be in ten years.

Exploring what psychologist Abraham Maslow called "peak experiences" is also helpful in tapping her core beliefs. Asking her about her most memorable life experiences will give you a clue as to what she seeks out of life—and what you can pretend to proffer her. Questions like, "When do you feel most beautiful?" "What was the happiest moment of your life?" "When were you most popular?" "What is the most exciting thing you have ever done?" are all a way of discovering her peak experiences. If she asks you why you are asking so many personal questions, simply tell her that you enjoy getting to know people on a deeper level and that she seems like a very interesting person, worth knowing on a more than superficial level.

You can also present this information exchange as a game, particularly if you are sitting at a restaurant table waiting for service. You can invite her to play the question game, "Have you ever . . . ?" or you can write down on a napkin "I feel excited when . . ." and hand it to her to finish. You can also simply offer to name all the things you like: "I like red sunsets, traffic-free tunnels, a smooth shave, warm sheets, cool pillows, broken-in jeans, and silk pajamas, what about you?"

If you don't feel comfortable asking her personal questions yet (or if she appears to be reluctant to reveal intimate information), you can always get her to open up by asking the "if" questions. Look around the place and say, "If you owned this place, what would you do to improve it?" or, while discussing the latest lottery winner, ask, "What would be the first thing you would buy if you won all that money?" You could ask, "What occupation would you choose if you didn't have to work for a living?" Or mention some of the places you plan to travel that summer, and then ask her, "If you could go anywhere in the world, where would you go?" You can also ask a general question such as "If you had magic powers, what would you do with them?" Finally, you can talk about some of your hobbies, such as sports, and if you find out that she doesn't particularly care for your hobby, you can jokingly ask her, "If I made you watch a hockey game with me, what would you make me do in return?" Think of yourself as an archaeologist of her soul who needs to gently unearth all of her core beliefs, bone by bone, without breaking any of them, then piece them together to figure out the skeleton of her worldview.

Daydream with Her

Once you find out her core beliefs and peak experiences, you can invite her to daydream together. Describe a special place to her that she would enjoy, then ask her to imagine it with you. Elaborate on the details, describing feelings and sensations. For example, if she mentioned how much she likes the beach, tell her that you would love to take a tropical vacation soon. Then say, "Wouldn't it be nice to jump on a plane right now and land on a deserted tropical island? We could kick off our shoes and take a walk on the beach, feeling the hot sand between our toes, watching the big red sun set as we sip our piña coladas to the cries of the seagulls. And then you and I could go dancing to reggae music all night and sleep in in the morning. I am getting sunburned just imagining it!"

Mirror Her Verbal and Nonverbal Language

While you are probing into her mind in an attempt to find out what her beliefs are, you can make her perceive you as similar by subtly echoing her words, way of talking, dialect, or body language. If she tends to say "I am fixing to leave," you can repeat that statement later in the night. The goal is not to sound like a parrot but to give her a subliminal feeling that you are like her.

Jargon to Use with Models and Actresses

HIT	MISS
Booking	Gig
Layout	Spread
Pictorial	Pictures
Centerfold	Fold out
Rehearse	Practice
Go-see	Interview

If she is a foreign hottie, you will definitely gain some points by knowing some words and phrases in her language. Don't worry, you don't have to learn a whole new language, just pick up some commonly used phrases. Even if you don't meet a hottie speaking that language, you can always impress your friends and all-American hotties with your erudite, worldly ways.

Qui vivra vera

Que será será

Joie de vivre

Magnifique

Bella

Wanderlust

Schadenfreude

Zeitgeist

Siesta

The nonverbal mirroring is even more important than the verbal one because it creates a sense of ease, comfort, and intimacy. When people are engaged in an interesting conversation, they often assume the same poses and make the same movements. They may lean in the same direction, or cross their hands in the same manner, and make the same facial expressions. Use mirroring to create instant rapport with her, unless you find it so distracting that you cannot focus on the conversation. In that case, mirror her only while she is speaking.

Highlight Complementary Differences

In addition to emphasizing similar outlooks, you should look for complementary differences that you may have with her. While opposites seldom attract when it comes to major issues—we are often attracted to those whose qualities complement our minor deficiencies. For example, I absolutely hate cooking and want nothing to do with the kitchen, yet I am definitely attracted to men who can cook. Why? Because if neither one of us can cook, then we'll either have to starve, hire a personal chef, or perpetually rely on takeout! As she talks about herself, confessing a deficiency in talent or ability, look for a way that you can fill in that gap in her ability. Women who are not good at managing money often look for a guy who is financially savvy. In addition, little differences can spice up a relationship and offer new ideas, but these differences have to be in *superficial* layers, such as hobbies and interests, rather than core beliefs, such as religion or philosophy of life. For example, she might find it exciting that you speak a foreign language that she does not, but she will probably find it off-putting if you are a hardworking, devoted Catholic while she is a hedonism-loving atheist. Similarity in views about relationships and family is particularly important. Penthouse Pet Aria Giovanni divorced her rock star husband because he wanted to have only one child with her, while she wanted at least three.

Occasionally, people crave to be with someone who is entirely different from him or her. These are often folks who are high in sensation-seeking traits and who want to experience something different because they are easily bored (I call them "novelty-experience collectors"). I knew one centerfold who wanted to experience having sex with men of as many different ethnicities as possible for the sheer thrill of comparison. One time we were out on a promotion, and a young man of Indian descent began talking to us. She whispered to me, "Oh, I have to hook up with that guy! I haven't been with an Indian man yet!" If you meet such a sensation-seeking hottie and you happen to be the missing collection item in her black book, by all means emphasize that difference! That guy actually blew it because he mentioned he was only part Indian and seemed to be uncomfortable with that part of his heritage. However, remember that such liaisons usually do not last and she is likely to move on to another missing item in her collection after you become a notch on her bedpost.

Use Small Talk as Transitions

A good conversation is like a radio show; it flows without long silences but with occasional interruptions for commercial breaks. Similarly, when a topic you are discussing comes to a logical conclusion and you don't know yet what to discuss next, you can take a break by engaging in so-called small talk. One of the best small-talk topics is popular culture. As I pointed out before, women in general—and hot women in particular—love to discuss celebrities (even educated and erudite women like me indulge in that guilty pleasure). I always look forward to catching up with my celebrity gossip when getting my routine beautification services such as manicures, pedicures, hair highlighting, and massages. Next time when you walk by a nail salon, peer inside and see what all those attractive hotties are reading—tabloids and celebrity gossip magazines, along with classic women's magazines. Most of these women would be happy to share their opinions with you about celeb news, such as wether or not Brangelina is going to get married. Beside celebrity gossip, most hot women will be happy to discuss the latest movies, fashion, popular music bands, top songs, and exotic travel locales. If you want to be facile in discussing these topics, subscribe to or pick up copies of magazines such as *US, People, Psychology Today,* and travel magazines. Some men swear by reading women's magazines, such as *Cosmopolitan* and *Vogue,* claiming they make them more able to understand women and be better conversationalists. You can use celebrity gossip to demonstrate the qualities that appeal to women such as kindness and magnanimity.

> YOU: That girl has Britney Spears' look. BTW, what do you think of her decision to cut off all her hair?
> SHE: That was crazy. I think she looks awful with that bald head.
> YOU: She must have been going through a lot of personal turmoil to do that.
> SHE: You feel bad for her, huh?

Some guys feel they have to talk the entire time. It is OK to have silent breaks, although it is important to distinguish when silence is meaningful and when it is awkward. You don't have to talk while you are studying the menu, eating, admiring a work of art, or listening to a song. That is why choosing restaurants with live entertainment (Russian restaurants are big on it, such as pianists or accordion performers) is always a good idea—you can always just turn to the performer and enjoy the music during pauses in your conversation. Some places such as nature walks lend themselves to silent observation. If you are waiting for service at a restaurant or in line to get in somewhere and you feel the silence is getting awkward, you can always do something playful, such as offer to read her palm or challenge her to a game of tic-tac-toe, hangman, or rock-paper-scissors. Tell her that you can deduce what her personality is really like from these games. One guy I dated took a napkin and poured some hot chocolate on it, then pressed it together, creating what looked like a Rorschach inkblot. He then proceeded to ask me what I saw in it, creating some lively discussion as a result. His tactic was particularly clever, because he was using a game to delve deeper into my psyche while drawing from the area I was interested in—psychology.

How to Tell That the Silence Is Awkward

• She is looking around the room uncomfortably

• She is avoiding looking at you directly

• She is picking at her food, pretending to eat

• She goes to the bathroom for the nth time

• She starts chatting with service personnel

Give Her a Unique Compliment

> *You have perfection about you. Your eyes have music. Your heart's the best part of your body. And when you move, every man, woman, and child is forced to watch.*
> —KEITH CARRADINE to LESLEY ANN WARREN in *Choose Me*

Hot women know that they are hot; thus you are unlikely to impress her by pointing that out to her. In fact, you might even offend her if you compliment her on something she considers to be obvious, or if your compliment is not strong enough (such as telling a beautiful model "you know, you are a pretty woman"—of course she knows!). Stay away from showering her with such banal compliments; instead, give her a few carefully chosen and unique compliments. If you can't think of unique terms to compliment her with, pick up a thesaurus and look up synonyms for *beautiful*, *hot*, and *sexy*. While you are at it, think of other descriptive terms that you often use, such as *smart* and *sweet* and look up their synonyms as well. Choosing unique words will show her that you are a connoisseur of beauty, the kind of man who has been around sexy women and can truly appreciate her unique and superior sex appeal.

Words to Compliment Her

HIT	MISS
Sizzling	Hot
Ravishing	Pretty
Alluring	Attractive
Striking	Great
Dulcet	Sweet
Scrumptious	Tasty
Elegant	Stylish
Brilliant	Smart
Exquisite	Beautiful
Exotic	Different

TIP #15: To maintain your mystique, reveal little about yourself and concentrate on talking about her. To delve deeper into her mind, reflect her statements and ask questions that emphasize her feelings. Look for commonalities, emphasize complementary differences, dream with her, and give her a unique compliment. ✦

Top 10 Things to Avoid Talking About on the First Date

1. Religion. Unless you are trying to seduce a nun by convincing her you are one of Jesus' secret progeny, stay away from this most unsexy of all topics. Do you really want to remind her of all those Sunday school prohibitions against premarital sex that she has worked so hard at repressing?

2. Politics. Unless you are in a crowd of political fellow travelers, this is another polarizing subject to stay very far away from. If she is indifferent to politics, it will bore her to pieces. If she is a strong supporter of the opposite party, she will think of you as dumb at best or an enemy at worst. Besides, do you really think any discussion of George Bush can lead to anything romantic?

3. Weather. Unless you are a tsunami survivor or a weatherman by profession or a tornado is headed your way, don't talk about weather. It's boring, geriatric, and anticlimactic!

4. Your childhood. Grown-ups talk about adult subjects, and spending lots of time discussing your childhood will betray your immaturity. She doesn't care at what age you were toilet trained, and if you tell her about being a Wunderkind, she'll wonder what happened to all that potential.

5. Your family. Unless you are related to someone she knows and likes, or you are a descendant of the Kennedys or Rockefellers, avoid bringing up your family on a first date. Dwelling on your parents will put you at risk of appearing "undifferentiated" and "enmeshed with your family of origin." You want her to think of you as a potential sexual partner, not somebody else's child.

6. Your exes. Women are catty and hate competition—past, present, or future. As far as she is concerned, she is the only woman you have ever been attracted to. She eclipses all of your prior encounters, and when you are with her, all others are dust. Need I say more?

7. Sex. If you bring up sex before she feels the urge to have it with you, she will consider you a lecherous pervert, or worse, a sexual predator. You do want to learn about her attitudes toward sex, but you have to tread carefully at first to avoid turning her off. Do you know any "good" sexy jokes?

8. Money. Talking about money is plain uncouth and tacky. If you discuss how much you have, you will appear a capitalist braggart who is obsessed with filthy lucre—like Donald Trump! If you complain how little you have, you will come across as a proletarian loser who will expect financial support. Either way, she'll consider you a materialistic moron for bringing up the Almighty Dollar.

9. Death. Unless she is a vampire or a goth-lover, avoid discussing any aspects of our mortality. It's morbid, and anything morbid is a downer. You want her to feel happy and eternal in your presence, with you being an important key to her eternity.

10. Your health history. If you are wearing a cast from some dramatic sports injury, it is OK to play it up. But otherwise avoid talking about your health history. And no matter how much something is hurting you, don't complain about pain. Women are evolutionarily programmed to be attracted to healthy, disease-free, robust male specimens. And men are supposed to be stoically indifferent to pain, at least on the first date!

Fourteen

Manners and Protocols:
Behaving on the First Date

*I went out with this one guy; I was very excited about it. He
took me out to dinner, he made me laugh—he made me pay.
He's like, "Oh, I am sorry. I forgot my wallet." "Really? I forgot
my vagina."*
                                            —LISA SUNDSTEDT

Your overall demeanor on the first date will be her ultimate litmus test of your acceptability as a date. Many hot women will
accept an initial dinner date from a guy because they want a free
dinner, but they use the first date to weed out potential suitors.
You need to come across as casually relaxed and project a detached
interest without a slightest hint of lust. Do not come across as
overly excited, even if she is the hottest woman you have ever been
out with, and try to curb your enthusiasm.

Before you leave your house, make sure that you are well
groomed and that you are dressed appropriately for the place you
are going. Make sure you have your mints, your wallet, your cell
phone, and directions to all of your destinations. Plan to arrive
about ten minutes early—running late will increase your anxiety

and nervousness, and getting there too early will leave you too much time to brood and ruminate.

When she arrives, smile and say hello. Many guys ponder as to whether they should kiss a woman on the cheek, give her a hug, or shake her hand at this point. The form of your greeting depends on the prototype you are trying to project. If you are trying to act detached and mysterious, you don't have to do anything but say "How are you doing?" with an optional light touch on her shoulder. If you want to come across as a relaxed and informal bohemian, then give her a light hug with a pat on the back. If you want to project a European bonhomie, then give her two kisses—one on each of her cheeks. I am very fond of guys who practice this European form of greeting, as it comes across as suave yet warm. It does, however, require some practice to carry out smoothly. The only gesture I find a bit outdated and thus slightly maladroit is a kiss on her hand—but if you are trying to project an old-fashioned gentleman, then you can adopt that gesture as part of your prototypical repertoire.

HIT	MISS
A touch on the hand or arm	A handshake
A light hug	A bear hug
A cheek peck	A hand kiss
A double cheek peck	A lip kiss
"I am glad we could meet up"	"I am so happy to see you"

Many guys also assume that modern women of today no longer care for the guy to act chivalrous. In fact, most women, no matter how liberated they are, appreciate courteous manners in a guy, and hot women are no exception. Even if you are trying to project a strong masculine bad-boy prototype such as an athlete or biker, opening the door for her will gain you points without detracting from your image.

You Should:

• Open the doors for her, particularly when entering establishments, and preferably when getting in/out of the car

• Help take off her coat

• Pull out her seat in the restaurant

• Let her order first

• Offer to let her taste and approve the wine

• Wait until her meal is brought to begin eating

• Leave a little on your plate

• Suggest a dessert

• Pay for her dinner

• Refuse to let her contribute a tip

• Let her walk on the inside on the street

• Take her arm when crossing the street

You Should Not:

• Insist that she order an alcoholic drink

• Insist that she order a dessert

• Offer to split a dessert

• Hold her elbow when helping her get in the car

Similarly, having basic dining finesse is particularly important when you go out with high-maintenance hotties who are used to dining in highbrow establishments. Knowing how to pronounce foie gras or duck a l'orange and following the basic etiquette, such as placing a napkin on your lap, will help you project worldliness and savoir faire. Many guys begin to panic when faced with an arsenal of cutlery and the watchful eye of an overly ceremonious waiter. A simple rule of thumb is to start off with the outer utensils and gradually use the utensils in the direction toward your plate. But don't sweat it if you accidentally grab the wrong fork; as long as you behave cool and in control, she'll hardly notice. What she will notice is you starting your meal before hers is brought, eating too fast, or loud chewing or slurping. Watch your posture—don't bury your head in your plate and don't talk with your mouth full. Remember to savor the meal, not devour it. And make sure to be courteous to the waiter or waitress, even if you feel that the service leaves more to be desired. I once went out with a guy who sent his dish back in a most obnoxious manner. Needless to say, that kind of cocky rudeness turned me right off. Finally, make sure to offer her a dessert, pay for the meal, and leave a tip of at least 15 percent (20 percent is preferred). Many hot women, including me, judge the guy by the kind of tip he leaves—and most hotties detest cheapness.

There are a lot of self-proclaimed dating gurus who advocate not offering to pay for a woman's meal or "going Dutch." Guys, FORGET this advice! No matter how broke, handsome, confident, or crazy you are, never, ever make a woman contribute to her first meal with you. Of all the models I have interviewed—and all the ones I have spoken with over a decade in the show biz industry—I don't know a single one who would ever date a guy who allowed her to pay her share on the first date. In fact, if she insists on paying for her share of the meal, that is a clear indication that she is not into you! Treating her to your first meal together does not mean you will continue to pay for her. Pay for her on the first date and, if you sense she is into you, use it to your advantage by offering to allow her to treat you to the next meal you have together— and leave it up to her whether she wants to go out, cook for you, or order in.

If you are taking her bowling or to play tennis, make sure to leave your competitive spirit at home. Think of her as you would your little niece—she is unlikely to enjoy playing with you if you win all the time, so a little giving in will go a long way. Letting her win will make her feel competent and good about herself, and your ability to take the loss graciously will score you points as well. Similarly, if she is a fan of spectator sports, and you plan to take her along to a game, make sure not to get carried away by the game to the point where you begin to ignore your date. And by all means, do not bring your buddies along to the game! Not only will you behave differently, less flatteringly, in their presence, she might end up liking one of them more than you!

TIP #16: For your first date, arrive on time, give her a light hug and/or cheek kiss. Make sure to observe basic manners, such as opening the door for her, and basic dining finesse. Pay for her dinner and leave a generous tip. ✦

Things She Will Evaluate You On

- Was he well dressed?
- Was he well groomed?
- Did he pick me up on time?
- Did he have good manners?
- Did he open the door for me?

• Did he talk at me?

• Did he engage me in conversation?

• Was he interested in my opinion?

• Did he notice how I looked?

• Did he compliment me?

• How did he interact with others?

• Did he make sure I had a good time?

• Was this date more about him or me?

• Did he make me feel like I owed him something at the end of the night?

• Did he expect that I would sleep with him right away?

• What did he do to annoy me?

• Am I attracted to him?

• Do I want to see him again?

HOW TO READ HER INTEREST IN YOU

Ask, and ask sexy. Say, "Can I kiss you?" or "I am feeling like we oughta take off all of our clothes, grind our genitals together for twenty or so minutes, then hop back in the shower for a rinse and some cunnilingus, then jump back in bed, eat some Ben & Jerry's Cherry Garcia and then maybe have another go at it. How are you feeling?"   —DAN SAVAGE

Every guy wants to know how he is doing on a first date, but it is definitely not cool to ask. Indeed, asking whether she is enjoying herself or "Is everything OK?" is extremely annoying, at least to me. You don't want to show anxiety and uncertainty; and while you can ask how she likes the food, or the ambience of the restaurant, or "objective" aspects of the date, you can't ask whether she enjoys being with you. So how can you tell if your mystifying, commonality-reinforcing, and intimacy-building tactics are really working? There are no surefire ways to tell, and all women are different in how they express or exhibit their interest in a man, but there are some clues that you can use.

The Eye Test

A woman who is interested in a man will usually spend a lot of time looking at him. She will meet your eyes when she is talking to you; when she looks away, she will catch glimpses of you out of the corner of her eye. Her pupils will often dilate as a sign of interest as well. The song "I Only Have Eyes for You" pretty much sums up a woman's reaction to being with a man she likes or her feelings when she is thinking of hooking up with him later. On the other hand, if she is constantly looking around at everything but you or when she consistently fails to meet your eyes when she talks to you, that is a pretty good sign that you are striking out.

The Smile Test

If she is having a good time, and if she likes you, she will be doing a lot of smiling. Women smile a lot with friends too. However, most women are good at faking smiles to cover discomfort, so this test is not as reliable as the eye test or some of the others. But if she is smiling or laughing a lot, and the smiles seem genuine—especially when she is looking at you—that is always a good sign. Her going out of her way to laugh at your jokes, particularly if they are not all that funny, is an even better indicator that she is into you.

The Appetite Test

Her eating manners are a good litmus test of her sexual attraction to you. If she barely touches her meal, picking at, rather than eating, her food, chances are her stomach is full of butterflies.[54] And when women want to make a good impression, they are careful about their eating manners. God forbid a piece of lettuce gets stuck in her teeth, or a string of spaghetti falls on her pretty blouse! And she may consciously or unconsciously fear that if she eats too much, her stomach might stick out and make her look bloated. If she is anticipating being kissed by you, chances are she'll stay away from any spicy, garlicky, or fishy foods. She is also likely to make a couple of trips to the bathroom to make sure she looks perfect and to reapply lipstick and other makeup. If, on the other hand, she is devouring everything in sight, chances are she is not really into you. However, do not consider her poor appetite alone as a sign of her interest in you. Some beautiful women are on perpetual diets, and others have eating disorders like anorexia and bulimia, so consider her appetite within the general context of the situation.

The Alcohol Test

If she eats little but imbibes a lot, that is a good sign. When a woman is not comfortable with a guy she will tend to drink as little as possible out of fear of losing control. When she feels safe and at ease with you she is more likely to get intoxicated and will not be worried that you will "take advantage of her." However, there is a Catch-22 here. If you would like her to get inebriated in order to make her more susceptible for a quick lay, you might mistake her slurred speech for an indirect invitation to her bedroom; on the other hand, she is trusting that you will not use her intoxication as an excuse to grope or screw her. For that reason, do not try to get her drunk, as that will only lead to misunderstandings later; moreover, if she senses you are doing it, it will automatically put her in a defensive mode and turn you into a reject in her date book. If, on her own, she asks for refills for her drinks, it might mean that she would like some action later—but you have to then become defensive and tell yourself that you are not going to move on her until the alcohol wears off.

As with the appetite test above, do not take her intoxication alone as a sign that she wants you. Some hot women have substance abuse issues and will get drunk merely because they do it all the time.

The Money Test

If she is offering to pay for everything, chances are she is not into you. Because there is an unspoken understanding that your paying for everything is a form of "copulatory gift," which is almost universal in all animal species, her offering to pay for your dinner, drinks, etc. is a form of rejection. She probably does not want to feel obligated to you and wants to put you in her "friends" category.

The Good-bye Kiss Test

A kiss is an application for a better position.   —JEFF ROVIN

The ultimate test of her interest is the kiss test. If she moves away from you quickly when you part, you probably have not made the impression on her that you want to have made. If she offers you her cheek, chances are she is not completely sold on you (but all is not lost, either). If she offers you her lips, you are in scoring position. It's up to you then, whether and when to drive in the runs.

HOW TO GET THAT GREAT KISS

For many guys, knowing when and how to get a kiss—and then more—from your dreamboat is a big problem. Most guys would like to be able to ask the simple question, Can I get a good-night kiss? But that is decidedly uncool. I had one date who tried to get me to give him a kiss by saying, "Oh, I forgot, I haven't kissed you yet." I thought that was totally presumptuous of him, so he only got my cheek for a split second. Just sticking out your "big fish lips," as Pet Julie Strain put it, is also a no-no; in Julie's case, it earned her date a door slammed in his face. But if you can't ask, how do you know when it is OK to initiate a kiss?

In part, you can have a pretty good idea by how she has responded on the prior tests above: lots of eye contact, smiles, picking at her food, etc. means your advance to the kissing stage will likely be welcomed. If you are unsure of her willingness, there are ways to give her the opportunity to signal her readiness. When you are ready to part, whether it is in your car or at her door, you will want to look her directly in the eyes with a smile and thank her sincerely for a great evening. If you have walked her to her door or car and have her hand in yours, or your arm around her, you can very gently steer her into a face-to-face position while you give her this message. If not, place your hand gently on her arm as you thank her. If she shies away from your touch or brushes it off, she probably is not going to allow a kiss. But if she moves toward you at all, or holds your gaze intensely, you know she wants to be kissed! It's all in her look and response to your touch. As 2006 Pet of the Year Jamie Lynn put it, "If I am looking into his eyes intently, then go for it, damn it!"

▸ *A man who can't kiss can't fuck.* —CYNTHIA HEIMEL

If you can't read her nonverbal signals, you can go ahead and ask her, but do it in a playful, teasing, rather than supplicating, way. You can say something to the effect of "You have great lips. They are begging to be kissed, aren't they?" or "This is when I turn into a prince if you kiss me!" Chances are she will either blush or laugh, either one of which is a sign for you to make your move.

You can also project your intent by saying, "Would you like to kiss me?" and unless her answer is a blatant no, you can assume she does. If she answers with a hesitant reply to the effect of "Oh, I am not sure," you can say, "Well, let's find out," and proceed.

Once you have the invitation, how do you accept it? Very slowly, looking into her eyes, bring her into your arms. Don't rush this! Prince Charmings in all the stories take eons to kiss their princesses, and this is a Prince Charming moment. If she only is willing to let you kiss her on the cheek, she will turn her head as you move closer; you'll have to be satisfied with that. But if she is ready to be really kissed, her arms will slide around yours and her lips will come into position almost automatically in response to you gently pulling her close.

Once your lips meet, make the kiss as soft, sweet, and short as you can. Not only I but also all of my centerfold friends really creep out when a guy starts tonguing right away or mashes lips as if he were trying to deflate them. If you feel her responding with a kiss of her own, you can increase the lip pressure in very slow increments until she either breaks the contact or ups the passion by using her tongue. Playmate Charlotte Kemp describes the perfect first kiss as "soft, pliable, passionate lips—not too aggressive, not too limp—wanting, not needing."

▶ *There are three kinds of kissers: the fire extinguisher, the mummy, and the vacuum cleaner.* —HELEN GURLEY BROWN

Be sure not to make the kiss last too long. You don't want to test how long she can hold her breath and you want her to look forward to more. As Julie Strain put it, make it "slow, easy, and gentle, not too long, leaving me wanting more." Krista Ayne likes it "slow and passionate," but don't try to wiggle your tongue like a madman or stick your tongue down her throat. Erica Ellyson wants it "not too sloppy; slow, sweet, and sexy." While most women will break off a kiss first if she thinks it too long, you shouldn't wait for her if it seems to be getting longer than you expected. You can keep hold-ing her and looking into her eyes. As my friend Pet Courtney Tay-lor put, "If I want more, I will pull him closer" and kiss him again. Otherwise, make it sweet and sexy, then let her go.

While we are on the subject of kissing—one of my favorite activ-ities!—let me share with you the most common mistakes men make when they kiss a woman. Mostly they involve trying to be too forceful and using too much tongue. As Pet Courtney Taylor describes it, the worst kissing is "too forceful kissing," like when he "stuck his tongue too far back and moved it really fast." Julie Strain, who never minces words, recites her litany of don'ts: "Don't stick your tongue down my throat. Don't bite or bruise my lips. And don't chip my teeth—they're porcelain veneers, for God's sake." Drooling or slobbering during a kiss are also the "kisses of death" as far as hot women are concerned. Erica Ellyson said she was "scarred for life" by one particularly bad kisser, "as he slob-bered all over me everywhere—it was worse than being licked by a dog!" Another Pet, Brea Lynn, described a similar experience where a guy "slobbered on me and did the 'fish out of water' thing" (referring to the "wide mouth bass" kiss). Jamie Lynn, the 2006 Pet of the Year, hated it when a guy "put it [his tongue] in there and drooled on me;" and Playmate Charlotte Kemp was disgusted when a guy used his tongue like a "tongue depressor, desperate, in my throat—Yuck!"

So a word to the wise: keep it sweet, gentle, romantic, and short enough to make her want more. That way you will get a lot more chances to demonstrate your kissing prowess.

TIP #17: To determine if she's into you, note whether she is gazing at you, smiling and laughing a lot, eating a little and imbibing a lot, or letting you pay for her. The ultimate test, however, is if she lets you kiss her. Always subject her to the kiss test. To see if she is amenable, suggest that she looks like she wants to kiss you. If she laughs, go for it. ✦

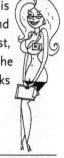

How to Get the Good-bye Kiss

HIT	MISS
Gaze into her eyes first	Surprise her
Compliment her lips	Ask her permission
Suggest she wants to kiss you	Suggest you want to kiss her

Worst Ways to Kiss

1. Sloppy chops. A kiss should be an erotic experience, not a gastronomic catastrophe. Too much salivation will make her want to look for that slurping, saliva-sucking device that dentists use. Make sure to breathe through your nose, and swallow from time to time so that you don't spray her with your spittle.

2. Deep-throat tonguing. Even if you have a long tongue, do not try to shove it as far down her throat as possible or use it to check out the cavities in her back teeth. Your tongue is not a slithering snake trying to unclog the sink, so keep it under control. There is nothing romantic about engaging her gag reflex, so keep the tongue action to soft, sensual explorations of her lips, tongue, and front teeth.

3. Head bobbing. If you want to be known as a lover and not a bob-blehead doll, try to hold your head steady while you kiss. Too much head weaving can put her at risk for a nosebleed or a chipped tooth. You should move your lips around to avoid "mouth mash-ing" and to give your kisses variety, but do it slowly and gently.

4. Mouth lock. Locking your jaw or stiffening your lips will make her want to use that car jacking device on you. Relax your jaw and keep your lips and tongue loose, as there is nothing worse than a tight-lipped kiss. Light, flickering kisses gradually increasing in intensity and passion do the trick, but always make sure that she knows you are a warm, romantic human being and not some cold-hearted robot.

5. Frozen lips. One kiss, however long, does not make you a Lothario. Variety is the spice of the amatory arts as well as in other aspects of life, so give her a series of different kisses, some short, some long, instead of one long, lip-locked kiss. Marathon kissing contests went out in the 1920s!

6. Wandering eye. Avoid looking around or checking out anything else other than her face while kissing her. If she's worth kissing, she's worth all your attention. You can either keep your eyes closed or dreamily half-open; if you opt for eye contact, avoid a wide-eyed blank stare. Gazing in her eyes can be a way to enhance intimacy, but make sure to blink from time to time.

7. Face licking. Only cats and puppies lick faces, so unless you are auditioning to be her four-footed pet, do not lick her face while kissing. Kissing her eyes, cheeks, and temples is nice, though, so don't be afraid to explore those areas with your lips. Just keep your tongue for mutual tongue kisses and she'll understand that you are a different kind of animal from her pet Fido. Save your licking expertise for all her down-under areas!

8. Tongue chewing. Unless you want her to run for the hills, avoid hard biting or chewing her tongue. If you are itching to use your teeth, you can nibble or gently bite her lower lip, which is supposed to have a direct connection to her clitoris, according to Tantric theory. But avoid crushing your teeth against hers.

9. Vacuum suction. She isn't kissing you to have her mouth vacuumed. You can gently suck on her tongue or lower lip, but avoid sucking so hard that she feels her mouth is being drained of all saliva or that her tongue is being pulled out.

10. Body stiffness. Even if your mouth is doing everything right, she will not be turned on if your body feels like a wooden statue. Use your hands to hug her, or to roam her body, to hold her face or chin, to caress her hair, or to squeeze her buttocks. Draw her close to you so that every inch of your body is against hers. Remember, you are a warm, affectionate, loving individual and not a cigar store Indian. Kiss like one!

Tip from the Scoring Experts *Giacomo Casanova, the legendary eighteenth-century Italian womanizer, dazzled women with his outrageous outfits, in brilliant colors and decorated with jewels. He was also highly intelligent, educated, and quick-witted; and he would regularly give gifts of jewelry and other items of adornment to the objects of his amorous quests. He also cultivated an air of femininity with his interests in clothes, theater, and domestic matters.*

Fifteen

Music and Poetry:
Getting into Her Panties

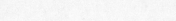

It is not enough to conquer; one must know how to seduce.

—VOLTAIRE

What happens after the first date depends on your intentions as far as your target hottie is concerned. If you are only interested in getting her into bed, you will want to use one set of strategies. But if you want her to fall in love with you, you will need to use a completely different approach. As you will see, these differing strategies are somewhat incompatible: if you conquer her quickly in the bedroom, you might not get her into a long-term relationship, while winning her love and adoration might require postponing sexual gratification. For that reason, this chapter and the next one follow two different tracks: one, for the direct route to a hot hook-up, the other, the more winding trail to a full-time lover.

How to Get a Shortcut into Her Pants

A woman's chastity consists, like an onion, of a series of coats.
—Nathaniel Hawthorne

Hot women may be harder to bed than the lesser variety—unless you are a multimillionaire willing to part with the hundreds of thousands of dollars some admirers have given centerfolds in exchange for sex. Don't doubt it: many of the hot women in the magazines or in show business are for sale for the right price. The trouble is that that price is out of league of most men. Plus, as soon as you stop the money flow, that's the last you'll see of those babes.

But don't despair. None of these centerfolds and glamour models that you see on the arms of rich "sugar daddies" are really into these men, and most of them have "real" boyfriends on the side. So your chances are not really diminished by their having wealthy suitors. Indeed, they might well get tired of servicing their, usually older and more demanding, patrons and be looking for some hot sex on the side.

What you need to show to them is that you can offer them something of value—whether material or intangible, something that will make them feel strong, positive emotions. Many women also need a strong justification to sleep with a guy on a first or second date. Below are some of the strategies you can use—just pick the one that works best with your talents and your prototype. By using these strategies, you are giving her an excuse to make an exception to her "no casual sex" rule. She needs to say to herself, *I could not resist him because he was so talented, so romantic, so special.* Remember, these do not guarantee you a fast score—they simply increase your odds with hot women that are easily seduced under the right circumstances.

If you have a thick wallet open it wide. Although most dating gurus are absolutely against buying women gifts in the first couple of dates, I am not quite so rigid. It is definitely not the best strategy if you intend to be dating her for a while, but if you are looking for a quick pathway into her pants, and your pant pocket is bulging with some spare cash—by all means, use some booty to get some bootie! Some guys enjoy buying women clothes and get quite turned on while watching them model sexy outfits! If you are into such a voyeuristic trip, do not be afraid to take her shopping. You can be innocuous about it and say something to the effect of, "A friend of mine gave me a gift certificate to Nordstrom, and I don't normally shop there, would you like to come along and help me spend it?" This has worked with me on a couple of occasions, especially the time when I agreed to accompany a man I'd just met to New York City's Henri Bendel and we ended up having sex in the store's fitting room! Of course, I hadn't intended to have sex with this guy—I hardly knew him; all I'd thought I was doing was agreeing to help him pick a new wardrobe for himself and get a few items for me in the process. He'd made it clear he wasn't expecting anything back, he just enjoyed buying beautiful things for beautiful women. But after I started trying on sexy lingerie in front of him, I found myself getting turned on, and before I knew it we'd been making out in the fitting room. I never saw that guy again because I was too embarrassed that I'd been such an easy lay for him—but I am sure he still smiles every time he walks by Henri Bendel!

If a hottie you have just met seems to be a clothing junkie, if her favorite pastime is shopping, and you have the money to spend, take her clothes shopping at a store of her choice, then insist on buying shoes to match the outfit she selects. Compliment her on how divine her body looks in the new clothes. Suggest she needs matching lingerie and take her to an appropriate store. When she tries on the lingerie, tell her she looks better than most Victoria's Secret models and deserves that million-dollar bra they sell every Christmas. Keep this up and those clothes will soon be on the floor next to your bed!

If you are a mover and shaker, let your body do the talking. Take her dancing—after all, it is one of the earliest precopulation rituals. You know what they say: dancing is a vertical expression of a horizontal desire. Slow dancing is the perfect way to build up her desire, so if you know a club that mixes slow and fast songs, by all means take her there. Although slow dancing may appear complicated, it is actually rather easy as long as you're not stepping on her feet. If you are a novice, stick with a simple side-stepping motion in which you and she both move clockwise. At the beginning of the dance, glance occasionally at the floor so that you can mirror her footwork, but don't stare at your feet. When you are stepping with your left foot, she will be moving her right foot, as she steps slightly backward, you will step slightly forward. Make sure that your feet do not lose contact with the floor, and if you constantly bump her feet, stagger your bodies slightly to the side so that the feet do not line up exactly.

With slow dancing you have to be bold yet sensuous, as well as attentive to her responses. Being too gentle and tentative might make you appear wimpy, while being too aggressive might frighten her. In short, she will deduce what kind of lover you are by the way you handle her during dancing. At the beginning of the dance, keep four to six inches' separation between your hips and your partner's hips and make sure your hips are directly above your feet. If she doesn't pull away, slowly move up closer. Because slow songs are usually played in pairs, you can always wait until the second song to pull her closer. If she acts uncomfortable or wants to sit down after the first song, she might not be a candidate for a quick lay. If she starts to rub your shoulders or back, move in closer and reciprocate with a gentle touch. Let your hands gently brush against her body, nuzzle your face in her neck. If she starts to grind against you, gently grind back. Take her hand and squeeze it gently but meaningfully. Gaze into her eyes and tell her you feel she is a kindred spirit and quite possibly a long-lost soul mate. You can continue making out once a fast song goes on or retire to somewhere more private for heavier petting.

Seducing through fast dancing is a bit trickier, as it naturally does not call for close body contact. Begin by dancing opposite from her, loosening your limbs, mirroring her movements, and gazing into her eyes. Then put one of your arms on her back and side and begin moving up and down. If she doesn't pull back, put your other hand on her and begin moving them up and down, but do not grope. At this point she will probably raise her hands and put them in her hair. At this point, slow down your pace—chances are she will slow down as well. Put your mouth close to her neck and gently breath around her earlobe and all around the neck area. You can also use one of your hands to pull back her hair and ever so gently touch her neck. You can then move your arms all the way up hers, pulling them up in the air and pulling her clothes. At this point, whisper sweet nothings in her ear, like "You are so sexy when you dance." You can also turn her around and pull her close to you, breathing on the back of her neck. The key is to build up her anticipation without being overtly and prematurely sexual. Physical exercise is an aphrodisiac by itself; coupled with some sexually suggestive gestures and romantic words, it may earn you a nice athletic bed bouncing!

If you can cook, use food to get her clothes off. This approach works best if you haven't taken her to dinner on your first date. Say you went to an amusement park and ended up munching some junk food there. Tell her that you will make it up to her by making her a nice dinner at your house for your next date. If she agrees to that, it is a good indication she wants to be seduced. Most women are charmed by men who can cook because it suggests a certain domesticity, appealing to their evolutionary desire for a man who will stick around and can feed their offspring, if need arises. Make her your favorite meal, and load it with foods that are natural aphrodisiacs. You can consult a cooking book such as *Inter Courses* for sexy recipes. Whether aphrodisiacs actually work or not is of little importance: because most people believe that they do, they work through the placebo effect. Serve the meal with her favorite wine. But don't attempt to get her sloshed—a little alcohol is a sexual disinhibitor, but a lot of alcohol is a ticket to a date rape charge. Follow the meal with her favorite dessert; here, think chocolate (which is full of PEA, a feel-good substance). Serve it with herbal tea (preferably mint to get rid of bad breath) and candlelight. Pick out the tastiest morsels and feed them to her; this approach, known as the "courtship feeding," is a shortcut to intimacy. Wish her "Bon appétit" and use other French words like "Voila!" I know it sounds really gay, but chicks really dig that stuff. Why do you think French guys have the highest frequency of sex in the world? Follow the meal by viewing suggestive films like *Like Water for Chocolate,* and *Chocolat.* With a warm full tummy and a buzz in her brain, your girl will soon be wanting a cuddle and more!

If you are an artist, whether professionally or at heart, use your artistic talent. Talk about your passion for artistic expression on the first date, and tell her you are looking for a perfect subject to inspire you. You can even show her some of your work, telling her that you have painted/photographed many gorgeous women in hopes of publishing a fine-art tabletop book—hot women are very competitive, and she will likely want to be part of that elite group of women. Offer to paint her portrait, and embellish it like crazy. Tell her that you really do think she is your long-lost muse, and when she is comfortable posing for you, offer to paint her a sexy lingerie full body shot (or a boudoir-style photo). Do not ask her to pose in the nude, as it will probably immediately put her on the defensive. Tell her she has to lay there really still surrounded by silk sheets and moonlight. Put on a light fan to blow her hair. Spray her body with light oil, taking care not to get it on the lingerie. Adjust the lighting and move the sheets for artistic effects while pretending not to be turned on. When she makes the first move, it is likely to invite you to join her on those silk sheets!

If you are a smooth operator, let your hands do the talking. Some guys are naturally great with their hands—they are what might be called the "touchy-feely" kind. If you are that kind of guy, engage in a nonsexual, nonthreatening touch from the first date. If she welcomes it and even reciprocates, she may also be the "touchy-feely" kind of girl. Not every person is comfortable with nonsexual touch. Whether you are or not probably depends on your childhood upbringing—whether your parents engaged in a lot of hugging and touching and encouraged you to do so as well. If she seems to act surprised by your touch, you can even explain this to her by saying, "I grew up in an affectionate family with a lot of physical contact." Chances are she will really like that statement because most women complain that men are not tender or physically expressive.

Remember, you want to come across as a warm and physical kind of guy, not a creep who cannot wait to get his hands on her. During conversation, reinforce positive messages with a fleeting touch on the hand. Use lots of "helpful" gestures such as brushing dust from her jacket or removing a stray eyelash from her cheek. If she looks tired or tense, offer her a foot, head, or shoulder massage. If your hands give her a warm, sensual massage (which you can learn to give in part 3 of this book), she will be ready for the next act.

If you have a great voice or can play an instrument, serenade her. No wonder Shakespeare wrote, "If music be the food of love, play on." If you can sing and/or play a musical instrument, you can invite her over to your house for a private concert you want to stage just for her. Start with light romantic ditties, and then move up to the more passionate tunes. Knowing how to shed a tear while singing a Ray Charles classic like "I Can't Stop Loving You" guarantees you to get laid—chicks love melodramatic stuff! Penthouse Pet Aria Giovanni said that she used to melt when she listened to her ex-husband play his music, and that was the main reason she married him.

If you and she are both sensation-seekers, take some risks. As I have mentioned in the section above, fear, anxiety, and uncertainty lead to an affiliative behavior (translation: she will end up in your arms). Heights, deep waters, and dangerous situations all cause that adrenaline rush that will rush her into your bed. Take her for a ride on a roller coaster or in a fast sports car or aboard a speedboat. Skydiving or scuba diving together are surefire ways to muff diving for those women who love thrills (just ask my sister, who had sex with her scuba diving instructor). Surprise also adds to the thrill. You can have your buddy pretend to go after her pocketbook and you can chase him away. (Just make sure there are no police around, or have some bail money ready.) When she's feeling that excitement, every woman loves to be held; and if you know how to use your hands on her body, you'll score!

If you have a silver tongue, it's as good as gold for enticing her into the sack. As Sganarelle said to Don Juan in Molière's *Don Juan:* "Well, what I have to say is . . . I don't know what to say; for you turn things in such a manner with your words, that is seems that you are right . . ." There is a well-known adage that the brain is our most important sexual organ, and your silver tongue is the key to her brain. If you can use words to make subliminal suggestions that will make her feel happy, warm, excited, relaxed, horny, and turned on, she will be yours for the taking. For example, if she is stressed out after work, tell her you can get her relaxed and happy with "progressive muscle relaxation," where you instruct her to tense and relax each muscle in her body, starting with her toes and ending with her facial muscles. As you encourage each one of her limbs to become warm, heavy, and relaxed, embed some hypnotic suggestions about the fire of desire that is energizing her body. Then add a visualization technique by asking her to conjure up a special place—a sanctuary—where she is floating on a cloud of ecstasy high above all earthly concerns . . . with you. The idea is to make her feel relaxed, happy, and turned on—

and to associate these feelings with you as the conduit for these emotions.

Some pickup artists have perfected the skill of the silver tongue by relying on subliminal messages to excite a woman. Ross Jeffries drew from a theory of neurolinguistic programming (NLP) based on underlying hypnotic language patterns to develop his theory of Speed Seduction (www.speedseduction.biz).* Using embedded commands and hypnotic suggestions, Jeffries developed a series of patterns that, he contends, can easily excite any woman, and even bring her to an orgasmic brink. These patterns are stories that describe pleasurable states of mind and positive feelings, such as the ones she would experience when dancing, listening to music, or eating strawberries and chocolate. In addition to describing these feelings of excitement, patterns also contain embedded commands that are supposed to focus her mind on what you are saying, such as "Focus on those feelings . . . surrender completely." Patterns also contain subconscious messages known as binder commands, such as "That's the way to do it. Now, with me, it's different because . . ." which should subconsciously be interpreted by her as "Do it now, with me" due to the subtle inflection used. Such a subliminal command, which Jeffries termed "thought binding," is supposed to bind her feeling of desire and arousal to you. Patterning also uses subtle sexual innuendos, or double entendres, such as "Create an opening for it . . . feel that thought penetrate you . . . you come over and over again to the same conclusion" to give her subconscious sexual suggestion.

*Used with permission of Ross Jeffries.

Double Entendre Phrases Used by Ross Jeffries

PHRASE	PRONOUNCED AS
These values are below me	Blow me
A feeling of happiness	Hap-penis
A new direction	Nude erection
The sky is so beautiful	This guy is so beautiful

Another important element of Speed Seduction is embedded commands and suggestions, which basically dictate to her how she should be feeling. Some feelings you can suggest directly, such as "Have you ever felt that wonderful feeling of wind in your hair?" or "Don't you just love slipping into the hot tub after a long day of work, feeling the heat working its way up your body?" The idea is to make her feel those pleasant emotions, and to subconsciously credit you with making her feel that way. However, you cannot be as direct when it comes to making obviously sexual suggestions. This is where you can utilize quoting, in which you present something as if it is coming from someone else. Here's an example from Ross Jeffries (www.speedseduction.biz):

> Some men are so crude. I can't believe what I saw this dude do the other night. He walked up to the girl sitting at the bar next to me and said to her, "Imagine us totally making out and you are getting so incredibly turned on by it. If you were to feel that right now, try not to think about me eating your pussy all night long and getting really horny." I can't believe a guy would ask a woman to think about it all night long.

If you have a good verbal memory and decent acting skills, you might want to check out Ross Jeffries' website and memorize some of these patterns. They provide a good backup plan for when you run out of conversational material and need to utilize something to keep her from getting bored. However, I don't recommend relying on them exclusively for getting laid, as you run the danger that some other guy has already tried to use the same pattern on her before. It is better to choose your favorite words and phrases from these patterns and to practice incorporating them into sexual double entendres when you are having conversations with hotties.

TIP #18: If you want to get her in the sack fast, you can try one of the following strategies. If you are well off, take her shopping; if you are a great dancer, take her dancing; if you have a musical or artistic talent, use it to seduce; if you are great with your hands, use your magic touch to give her a massage; or, if both of you are sensation-seekers, take some risks with her. Finally, if you have the gift of gab, use the power of your words to make her feel horny. ✦

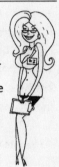

Myth Rebuffed: HOT WOMEN GET TURNED ON BY SUBTLE PUT-DOWNS OR "NEGS."

This approach, propagated by Mystery, a famous pickup artist, is supposed to be used only on perfect 9's or 10's. It's grounded in the faulty belief that gorgeous women are overly confident and do not respond to compliments, thus the way to get their attention is to pretend that you are not that interested and that you are "qualifying" her by making a subtle insult disguised as a compliment. Examples are: "Nice nails, are they real? No? I guess they look good anyway" or "You blink a lot" or "Funny how your nose wiggles when you talk." Mystery claims that when he uses these kinds of statements on gorgeous women they respond by working harder to gain his attraction. Let me tell you—this is total bullcrap! For me, these kind of petty, immature statements would suggest that a guy is a total weirdo or some strange fetishist. In fact, it would be an instantaneous turnoff! And all of the centerfolds I have interviewed wholeheartedly agree.

Top 10 Traits of a Girl Who Goes for One-night Stands

1. She dressed provocatively. If she's showing you a lot of tits and ass, she likely wants to do something with it.

2. She wears a lot of makeup. Makeup, particularly bright red lipstick, is often used to signify sexual availability.

3. She is well educated. Women with higher education have been found to have a greater number of sexual partners. Why do you think men love girls who wear glasses?

4. She has recently broken up with her ex. A woman on the rebound is likely to be seeking new affirmation of her attractiveness, and sex is the best one there is.

5. She is an atheist or agnostic. If she is not afraid of the Wrath of God, she is more likely to let go and have fun. Religion is generally a sexual inhibitor and best confined to committed relationships.

6. She is independent and aggressive. Studies have reported that independent and aggressive women have more sexual fantasies; and the more the merrier when you are looking for one-shot sex.

7. She is from a liberal family. Guilt about sex has its origins in a sexually restrictive and punitive upbringing (see number 5 above for further confirmation).

8. She is ovulating. Women are often hornier in the middle of their cycle, and more likely to cheat on their spouses. How would you know she is ovulating? Studies have shown that men may be able to perceive female genital secretions called ovulins, which are only released during ovulation!

9. She is a passionate dancer. Dancing has been defined as "a vertical expression of a horizontal desire." Or, putting it another way, if you find your arms full of ripe, undulating fruit, it is time for a snack!

10. She is a hedonist. She believes that life is too short, so why not carpe diem, or more precisely, carpe nochem?

Myth Rebuffed: HOT WOMEN ARE REALLY SELECTIVE IN CHOOSING WHOM THEY SLEEP WITH.
This is definitely not true. Hot women, on average, tend to be more promiscuous than less attractive women. They invest a lot of time, effort, and money into maintaining their sex appeal, and they like to show off their bodies. They tend to be more exhibitionistic, narcissistic, and impulsive, and constantly desirous of affirmation of their sex appeal. For all these reasons, they are actually easier to bed than average women, provided you offer them something of value or something that promises them pleasure.

Sixteen

Beyond Pavlov and Skinner: Getting into Her Heart

It is easy to show that the value the mind sets on erotic needs instantly sinks as soon as satisfaction becomes readily obtainable.

—SIGMUND FREUD, *Sexuality and the Psychology of Love*

You don't get high-quality sex without love.

—DR. ALEX COMFORT

If your goal is not simply to bed a hot woman but to get her to fall for you, your strategy needs to be more complex than the ones used to maximize your chances of getting laid. Robert Greene emphasizes the importance of taking your time if you want your quarry to fall in love with you. "Seduction is a process that occurs over time—the longer you take it and the slower you go, the deeper you will penetrate into the mind of your victim . . . By taking your time and respecting the seductive process you will not only break down your victim's resistance, you will make them fall in love."[55] Many men who make it past the first date and seem to have a woman's interest let their guard down and begin to "pursue" a woman. This is a big mistake and often leads to her losing interest in him, sometimes before she ever sleeps with him, and sometimes right after. So how do you get her to crave more and more of you?

The formula is actually rather simple: **yearning = anticipation of a reward, spiced with mild frustration.** We tend to crave things that make us feel good, things that we look forward to getting because we do not get enough of them, and things that we never know whether and when we are going to get again. Take a simple example of your favorite food. For me it is chocolate-covered almonds. Not only do I love the taste of them but chocolate also contains PEA, a feel-good chemical. No wonder I get a druglike withdrawal when I don't get a dose of them for a long time. Having a couple of chocolate-covered almonds always makes me crave more; however, when I eat a whole bag of them, I feel satiated and no longer crave them for a while. The same principles apply to people—we like to see those folks who make us feel good on a regular basis but usually grow bored and tired of them if we see them too often. The key is to get her to experience feelings of pleasure and enjoyment while in your company, peaking her anticipation by keeping your meetings and the rewards you give her exciting and unpredictable, while at the same time leaving her a bit frustrated by being sometimes unavailable. By rationing your enjoyable presence, you will make her crave you, the way I crave those chocolate-covered almonds. Here is how you do it.

Take Charge

Women love strong, determined, dominant, decisive guys who can take control and lead the way. Use every situation to show her that you are in charge and can take care of her. Don't ask her "What do you want to do today?" Keep her guessing and surprise her with well-thought-out entertainment, whether it's a fancy restaurant, tickets to the circus, or a picnic in the park. Since you now know more about her, and learn more with every date, you can plan these entertainments with even more confidence, knowing what is likely to be perceived by her as fun, exciting, and romantic.

Some of the ways you take charge do not involve dates, as much as they do making yourself indispensable to her happiness. If she tells you her car is giving her problems, you show up on her doorstep with your tools and either fix the problem or take it to the garage and get it fixed. Whether it be a stopped-up kitchen sink or difficulty in getting an insurance claim paid, offer to solve the problem for her. You are now turning her everyday life into one in which you seem to be indispensable, and that will make her start to believe that you might be a lifetime "fit."

Keep Control of Your Emotions

In addition to being "in charge" of planning dates and helping her with problems, you have to be in charge of yourself. Men often lose all self-control in the presence of hot women, appearing too eager, too needy, or too dependent on their approval. This can be disastrous with a beautiful model-type who has had tons of guys panting for her panties. So, at all times, it's important not to become emotionally invested in the outcome of any date. Do not allow her to reschedule your date last minute for no good reason or to blatantly flirt with another guy while out with you. Control your emotions, whether they are feelings of admiration, jealousy, embarrassment, or anger. Be prepared to walk away from her if she is not behaving in a way consistent with your self-image of a confident, popular leader.

This is the hardest thing for a lot of guys to do, but it is among the most crucial things if you want to really win her heart. She wants a man that *she* can be emotionally dependent upon, not some wimpy guy who is constantly worried about his status in her life or is frequently angry, sad-faced, or uncommunicative. Staying in control applies to not only your emotions toward her but also how you behave with others in her presence. Why is James Bond so attractive to all those hotties? He is always in control, resourceful, and levelheaded, even when whole armies of baddies have him surrounded. Learn to act with Bond-like cool in her presence, no matter what you feel inside—and if you do it constantly, you will soon *be* cool quite naturally.

Limit Your Physical Presence

"Let there be spaces in your togetherness," advised Kahlil Gibran. One of the main mistakes that men make with beautiful women is giving them too much affection and attention too soon. While you might feel like seeing her every day, remind yourself of the wisdom of the old proverb "Absence makes the heart grow fonder." Have you ever had so much of your favorite food that it no longer tasted good—perhaps to the point where you developed an aversion to it? On the opposite extreme, have you ever tasted something so delicious that you wished you could have more? Romantic interludes are like caviar—they're best appreciated in small doses.[56] Moreover, we always want more of what we cannot possess, or at least immediately possess. For all of these reasons, it is important to "give her the gift of missing you," or, as Julie Strain puts it, "Make me miss you. Don't just add Julie and stir."

By that Julie and I mean limit your physical—but not emotional—presence in her life. Try not to see her more than once or twice a week at the beginning, but do not let more than a few weeks go by between your meetings. If you think she is beginning to take you for granted, have a project out of town that will keep you away for a few weeks. Never leave her satiated with your being around. Give her the sweet torment of yearning for you. When she tells you she misses you, you know you are on the right track—be sure to reciprocate, as you never stop pointing out commonalities in your feelings. There is a French proverb: "Ces sont les petits separations qui entretiens les grand passion"—"It is little separations that maintain great passions."

Stay Connected

This is an important point. To make her yearn for your physical presence, consistently remind her of how fun you can be by leaving occasional phone, e-mail, and text messages. Remember the other adage: "Out of sight, out of mind." While you are out of her sight, make sure you stay on her mind. Call when you promise to call—you want to appear unpredictable, but *never* unreliable. When you give her gifts, make sure they remind her of you—whether it is a memento from your date, a photoframe with a picture of her favorite singer with your voice recorded on it, or some other original "personalized" gift.

Look, you're going to miss her too, yearn for her even—why else would you be pursuing her for a long-term relationship? But you can't let that yearning crack the image of the Prince Charming you are building in her mind. So use your yearning time to plan your next surprise date or gift or call. Remember: you are in charge! She has to sit home and wonder what you will do next, when you will want to get together again, while you have the advantage of knowing what you are planning and preparing for just when those events will occur. Use that advantage to keep yourself ever in her mind, while never letting her think she is calling the shots.

Give Her Symbolic Presents

A lot of so-called dating experts advise guys against giving any presents to a woman they are dating because doing so would suggest that you are "buying" her attention. Big mistake! Women, particularly beautiful women, love receiving gifts. The key is to know when and what kinds of gifts are appropriate. Stay away from expensive, impersonal presents like jewelry and gifts that are too clichéd—instead of giving her red roses for her birthday, get her some pussy willows or wildflowers. Presents should be small tokens of your affection for her—cards, bookmarks, self-made crafts, and souvenirs from places you've traveled to. The message of your gifts should be "I took the time to think of you" and "When you are good to me I reward you with tokens of my attention and affection" rather than "I have to give you gifts to get love or sex in return."

You can also use gifts to keep her sexually turned on and keep sex on her mind. If you are good with a camera and Photoshop, offer to take some sexy lingerie shots of her, then frame the best one and give it to her. This way every time she looks at that photo she will think of the great sex you had right after it was taken. If you like a particular perfume on a woman, get it for her and insist that she wear it when you make love—this way every time she puts it on, she will think of you. Body lotions and massage creams make great gifts because they feel the best when someone else (read you!) applies them. On a special occasion, you can buy her a lingerie piece or a sexy pair of heels and tell her you want to see her model them for you. I once dated a guy with a foot fetish, and he frequently brought me pairs of sexy (albeit inexpensive) strappy sandals. Although I knew he was really buying them for himself because my putting them on turned him on, I always looked forward to seeing him—and I never knew when he would bring a new pair of sandals, because he used variable interval reinforcement (see below), cunning man!

Ask Her for an Occasional Favor

Occasionally, ask her to do you small favors, such as pick up a paper for you, purchase movie tickets, or make a reservation. She will be more likely to fall for you if she invests some effort in having a relationship with you than if you do everything for her all the time. Research has shown that people tend to value and appreciate things more when they cost them effort or money. If something is free, we tend to consider it junky. Similarly, when we put ourselves out for a cause, we tend to consider it a worthy cause.[57] If we find ourselves doing things for another person that are not in themselves rewarding, we are likely to conclude that we must really like that person—otherwise, why would we do it?

When a hot woman catches herself doing something for you, she must justify in her mind the reason she is doing it. If she can't rationalize why she is going out of her way to do something for you, she would experience cognitive dissonance, or mental conflict. So she tells herself that she must really like you, otherwise she would not be doing this unrewarding task. So whenever she does something for you, do not be overly grateful—act like it is perfectly natural for her to do you a favor or give you a gift from time to time, because you are her equal and are perfectly worth it. Obviously, don't overdo asking for favors, or you will come across as a demanding jerk.

Do Not Be Overly Apologetic

I have a good friend who has a pathetically poor record of being mistreated and dumped by women despite the fact that he showers them with presents and does everything for them. This poor guy is a loser because he hasn't learned that giving women expensive gifts on every date and constantly apologizing for everything that might not go right with a date doesn't make him appear strong and in control. While it is a good idea to apologize for a major faux pas, such as being more than ten minutes late to a date, there is no reason to apologize for little things, such as not finding a parking space right by the theater, or the restaurant being out of their daily special. When it comes to things out of your control, such as a cancelled performance, no apology is ever appropriate. My friend, on the other hand, apologizes for everything. He apologizes when he could not get to the phone in time, when his date doesn't like her dish at the restaurant, and when she says she is not feeling well. Remember, princes don't apologize unless the issue is big enough to involve affairs of state; and you want to be her prince.

Create Positive Associations

You have probably heard the expression "salivating like Pavlovian dogs." In the famous experiment, Russian psychologist Pavlov rang a bell at the same time as he offered his dogs food. Soon the dogs started to salivate at the sound of the bell, even without the food. Pavlov created what is called "a conditioned response," or created association between a feeling and a neutral object. You can probably remember salivating for your favorite ice cream at the mere sight or sound of an ice-cream truck.

Similarly, you can create positive associations in your interactions with your hottie. For instance, every time she feels happy or laughs or enjoys some pleasurable activity with you, you can touch her in a specific place, such as an arm or shoulder, and say something like "I love to see you happy." After repeated pairing of her feeling happy with your touch, you have created a conditioned response. Now, when she is feeling down, touch her in the same place, and say the same phrase. Doing so should evoke happy feelings in her. But do not overuse this technique—if the ice-cream truck was always out of your favorite ice cream, you would eventually stop getting excited at the sight of it.

Creating memorabilia, or souvenirs, from your dates is another way to build such positive associations. Just having a framed picture of you and your honey at the amusement park on her mantelpiece will be a constant reminder to her of the fun you had—and of you! Part of staying connected is to have these positive associations constantly in your girl's memory. To again quote *The Art of Seduction*, "The gifts you give and other objects can become imbued with your presence; if they are associated with pleasant memories, the sight of them keeps you in mind and accelerates the poeticization process."[58]

Reward Only Desirable Behavior

This reward principle is based on B. F. Skinner's operant conditioning. By rewarding desired behavior in a step-by-step escalation, you can train a bear to dance or an elephant to roll over (in animal training this is called "shaping"). But as Skinner proved with his boxes, you can train people this way too. You may want to "shape" your honey to behave more in the way you desire. For example, if the object of your affections tends to vacillate between sweetness and bitchiness, reward her behavior only when she sounds sweet and is demonstrating the attitude you like. By "rewards," I don't mean you have to give her gifts every time she acts sweet to you and cooperates with your plans. The rewards I am referring to in this case are intangible, like approval, admiration, and affection. For instance, if you call her to ask her on a date and she answers in an irritable voice, "Oh, it's you. I am in a rush right now, what do you want?" it's time for some "shaping." Instead of saying "Oh, I am sorry, I'll call you back later," tell her "Call me when you are not in a rush" and hang up. Do not call her again until she has called you back. When she does call you, if she still sounds irritated, tell her "I am in a rush right now and will call you back in a few hours." In this way you are not reinforcing disrespectful behavior.

When she shows up on time and looking great, reward her with a smile and a compliment, and tell her you have a special surprise for her for your next date—you are getting tickets to her favorite show. If she subsequently acts bratty, act cooler to her and call her later that evening and tell her you were not able to get the tickets. Whereas you don't want to declare to her "I am not taking you to the show because you acted like a bitch," subconsciously she will get the message that you will not go out of your way to please her unless she pleases you. Remember, withdrawal of a reward (whether it is a promise of something tangible, attention, or affection) is also equivalent to punishment, which is an effective behavioral modifier. The important thing is to "punish" or reward the behavior shortly after it occurred, as delayed punishment or reinforcement is not very effective because it is hard for her to make an association between the two.

Use Variable Reinforcement

Slot machine designers know how to get you hooked on their one-armed bandits. It's called "variable interval reinforcement," and it involves programming the machines to produce just enough of a return to keep the customer excited and playing but not enough to get him bored or satiated. You can hook your honey by using this same principle. Don't give her gifts and compliments every time, only sometimes, and make those times variable, so she never knows when she might get one. When you reward her only irregularly, but often enough that she never forgets getting these rewards, she will develop anticipation for each of your meetings: "Am I going to get lucky and get a special gift today?" and extra excitement when you do reward her. You can combine this same principle with shaping to further influence her behavior. You do that by increasing the behavioral standard required to "earn" a reward. For example, you might memorialize your first public kiss in a photo or souvenir (girls get incredibly romantic about guys who even remember when they first kissed, much less where and under what circumstances). But before you give her another such memento, you would require that she go much further, like some hot makeout in a theater or restaurant. Each "raising of the bar" can be made a step on the progression you have in mind for her.

Tap into Her Unfulfilled Wishes

Every person has an unfulfilled wish, a secret desire, or a deep-seated insecurity. As I mentioned before, beautiful women are often insecure about their looks, and all of us have wishes and desires that we are not willing to share with everyone. These insecurities, as well as her unrequited longings, are your opportunities. Find her secret craving and fulfill it; all of a sudden you'll rocket to the top of her date list—all the more so if her craving is sexual in nature. Help her get over her insecurities by showing that you like her the way she is. For example, I always have been a bit paranoid about my waist size, as it isn't as Barbie-like as some models' waists. However, one guy really won my affections by telling me he liked women with long legs and short torsos. So if you learn the things that worry her, make it a point to be her main source of reassurance.

Be Affectionate

Most guys think that being confident translates into acting macho—haughty, standoffish, unaffectionate, and emotionally unavailable. In fact, hot women fall hard for men who are both strong and sensitive *and* who shower them with affection. Many men are afraid to be physically demonstrative with a woman for fear that public displays of affection will make them appear to be wimpy and supplicating. But truly smooth operators know how to utilize affection as the ultimate weapon in their women-getting arsenal of tricks. Every woman craves tenderness and affection because women produce greater amounts of the "warm and cuddly" hormone oxytocin in response to physical closeness—which is the reason why so many women will seek out sexual encounters in order to receive intimacy and closeness. Getting her high on oxytocin by showering her with affection when you are physically with her but rationing your physical presence is the ultimate hook. Being affectionate + elusive = obsession. A famous Russian poet, Anna Ahmatova, wrote that "tenderness can turn women into beggars and slaves."

Conceal Your Lust

Nothing is more unappealing to a beautiful woman than a guy who appears too horny and eager to get her in the sack. "I hate it when a guy is salivating at the mouth like a rabid dog," said one of the models I interviewed. You should not act asexual and uninterested, but your lust should be well controlled under your guise of a man who has had plenty of sexual satisfaction. James Bond is attractive to women precisely because he acts so cavalierly toward their charms, secure in the knowledge that he can get sex from many other women any time. A man who acts this way is a challenge, even to a hot model, as she will think that if you aren't groping her, you must be groping some other chick. That will get her competitive instincts engaged, and she might want to increase the sexual heat in her behavior to get you lusting more openly for her—which is exactly what you want, right?

Build Up Sexual Tension

Directly propositioning a woman is a bad move. Most women have issues with overtly admitting their desires for sex, and social mores lead them to turn down any proposition that might suggest that they are whorish or of "loose morals." Society tells a woman that she has to put up a chase, so she wants to be seduced, to have her reluctance overcome with overwhelming desire for her man. This means you have to be more subtle in eliciting her desires, building sexual tension during the date through eye contact, sexual innuendos, and nonsexual touch until she is turned on and ready to put matters into your hands quite literally. Throughout your dates with her, discreetly and fleetingly touch her hands, arms, shoulders, back, and face. Avoid grabbing her breasts or any body part with an obvious sexual connection, but a brush of your hands across her chest as you help her on with her coat, for example, is perfectly acceptable. These "accidental" touches can be upgraded as the relationship progresses, but the object is to indirectly get her to think of sex.

Delay Having Sex with Her

You might think this is absolutely crazy advice—why would you go through all the trouble of pursuing a woman if you are not going to have sex with her? However, this is just another example of how denial increases desire, as we discussed earlier; and your ultimate goal is not to deny her intercourse altogether but to make her wait for it. Then, when you do "consent" to doing her, you win not only her body but her heart and mind as well.

In psychology, this phenomenon is called *reactance* (lay folks use the term *reverse psychology*). Reactance is defined as wanting to do the exact opposite of what you are compelled to do. Playing "hard to get" evokes our feelings of reactance. When we are denied something we believe is due us, we end up desperately wanting it. Beautiful women are used to feeling sexually irresistible and to seeing men being overcome with desire and losing all control in sexual situations. However, meeting a man who can turn her on and please her while willfully delaying his own gratification is extremely impressive to a woman.

If delaying release becomes unbearable to you, you can allow yourself to have oral and manual sex with her, but not intercourse. You need to act like having intercourse with you is a special prize that you bestow only on a very special woman—and she needs to deserve it by showing you that she is worthy of it. The longer you put off having sex with her, the more she will want you. In addition, by doing so, you become a challenge to her—something most hot women are not used to. If she tries to push you toward intercourse, tell her to slow down because you are not ready.

I will never forget one of my first lovers, who drove me absolutely crazy by declining to have intercourse with me. He would kiss me, touch, fondle, and caress me for hours, until I would have several manual orgasms, but he would stop short of penetrating me. When I would practically beg him to penetrate me, he would insist that he was not ready and that we needed to wait to experience this ultimate act. I began to wonder whether he was saving it for another woman. This drove me crazy, to the point where I wanted to rip his clothes off and rape him—which I eventually did!

Combine the building of sexual tension with intercourse withholding, and you will have a powerful love cocktail. A date full of happy feelings and rising sexual tension, but the denial of a release, will cause her to want to see you again soon. But of course, you will vary your dating schedule with her to keep her off guard, thereby further increasing her tension and desire. All of these techniques are designed to be used together to create a crescendo of desire in her mind.

TIP #19: To get her to yearn for you, build up her anticipation with some mild frustration. Act busy, take charge, control your emotions, limit your physical presence but stay connected, give her symbolic presents, ask her for an occasional favor, create positive associations, reward her desirable behavior, ignore the undesirable behavior, use variable reinforcement, do not be overly apologetic, tap into her unfulfilled wishes, conceal your lust, delay having intercourse with her, build up sexual tension, and be affectionate. ✦

HIT	MISS
Court	Pursue
Keep in touch	Stalk
Empathize	Reveal your feelings
Expect reciprocity	Sacrifice your interests
Be sensitive	Be submissive
Ask for a favor	Burden with requests
Be polite	Apologize all the time
Act affectionate	Act clingy or mushy
Display interest	Display lust
Delay intercourse	Delay sexual touch
Miss her	Pine away
Seek agreement	Seek approval

TIP #20: If you find yourself falling for her before she is able to fall for you, you need to make a list of all her physical and character flaws and all the ways in which the two of you would not be compatible, and recite this list regularly. Force yourself to go out and date other women, as getting laid is the best antidote. Do not masturbate to her mental images—channel your passionate angst into a creative outlet. If your mood is predominately despondent, get a prescription for an antidepressant. ✦

Six Signs She'll Be a Dud in Bed

As you are falling for her, your mind is concocting daydreams of perfect togetherness. You imagine how wonderful it would be to make love to her for the first time. Yet the reality of being with her might be quite different from your fantasy, particularly if you overlook one of the signs below.

Telltale sign #1: obsessive squeamishness. If she is one of those obsessive-compulsive types who makes a bib for herself out of a restaurant napkin, pulls out antibacterial soap after each handshake, or runs to floss her teeth after every milkshake, chances are low that she will get down and dirty in bed. Who wants a girl who worries about you spilling your seed on her silk sheets? Or worse yet, crinkles her nose when you approach her mouth with your throbbing member? Or knows the exact number of germs exchanged during a kiss (a couple thousand, to be exact). Good sex is messy, and those who are too squeamish to get sweaty, smudged, and stained suck in the sack.

Telltale sign #2: rigid conservatism. If she dresses in gray suits and button-up blouses, wraps her hair in a bun, believes that liberal attitudes are ruining this country and that porn is the source of all evil, and, in her spare time, volunteers for the American Family Values Association, forget about her. You'd probably have to marry her even to get a good look at her pussy; and then all you could expect is that she would lay there in the missionary position and let you do her once or twice a month. She would rather get a root canal than step out of her sexual comfort zone, and if you try talking dirty to her, she'll report you as a sexual pervert. Here's a quick test to weed out these right-wing Ice Queens: leave a copy of *Penthouse*—or better yet, *Penthouse Variations* or *Letters*—out on your coffee table and watch her reaction. If she expresses shock, dismay, or distaste, just show her the door.

Telltale sign #3: religious dogmatism. Her middle name is Chastity, and she is serious about interpreting the Book literally. Chances are she has never masturbated and believes in procreative-only sex. Due to her convictions that premarital sex is sinful, you will probably never get past a dry-hump—and it'll be the worst one you've ever had. Even if she does let you proceed further, her subsequent shame and guilt will make you repent and regret every second of your sexcapade. So unless you are seeking spiritual enlightenment through shagging sexual martyrs, drop this one at her first quote from the Book.

Telltale sign #4: lethargic passivity. She is so passive that she not only lets you plan your every date but also insists you order for her from the menu. When you ask her about her sexual preferences, she responds with a spacey "whatever." She is constantly dazed and confused, and she would rather chill or get high than expand any kinetic energy—and that includes sexercise. Whether her lackadaisical attitude is pharmaceutically induced (downers or excessive pot smoking) or a dispositional laziness, you will be sick of initiating sex and orchestrating every sexual encounter—unless you are into having sex with blow-up dolls.

Telltale sign #5: excessive timidity. She blushes for any reason, has a nervous tic, and her nails are chewed up to the bone. When you take her to eat, she barely picks at her food out of fear that a piece can get stuck in her teeth. She fidgets anxiously when any sexual topic comes up, and chances are she clams up when it comes to discussing her past (non)experience in bed. Even if she does agree to do the nasty, she'll expect you to turn off all the lights and will require copious amounts of lubricant to get over the vaginal dryness caused by her shyness. And her nervous giggle when you try to open her tightly closed thighs will be the icing on this mood-killer of a cake. All you can hope for from this babe is that she has a slutty sister.

Telltale sign #6: narcissistic self-absorption. Her vanity has no boundaries as she checks and rechecks herself in the front mirror of your car. Everywhere you take her she has to make a grand entrance, showcasing her designer clothes and the latest Manolo Blahnik shoes. Your role is to continuously validate and glorify her—so don't expect some hot action from this cool cat. She might graciously condescend to enjoy herself while you are going down on her, but she won't deign to reciprocate. Instead, she will be too busy making sure her hairdo remains perfectly coiffed and her fake lashes are in place, and, while you are screwing her from behind, she will be checking out her manicure, to make sure none of it chipped from unscrewing that darn designer lubricant. Too much self-love makes for a lousy lay.

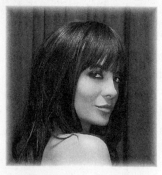

2007 *Pet* of the Year Runner-up Krista Ayne is usually attracted to artsy guys. "I've dated musicians, models, actors, and I've recently started dating a designer."

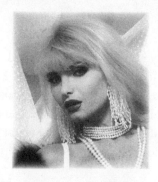

June 1994 Penthouse Pet Taylor Wane is most attracted to a guy who is a bit of a bookworm. "When I was a teenager I trained to be a schoolteacher, so I love long, in-depth conversations about history, the world, politics, food, anything! Exploring the mind is a powerful aphrodisiac."

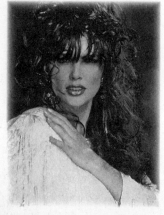

1993 *Pet* of the Year, Julie Strain has had long-term relationships with a bodybuilder, a Hells Angel, a comedian, and a comic-book artist, and has dated men from a variety of professions. She knows immediately when she finds what she likes: "My current husband and I moved in together on the first date."

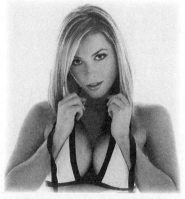

2007 *Pet* of the Year Heather Vandeven has dated everyone from musicians, businessmen, doctors, and an actor or two, but really likes a sweet, good-hearted artist. "Sometimes they don't have much money, but they make up for it in depth of spirit."

PART 3

Crossing Home Plate, or How to Bed Her

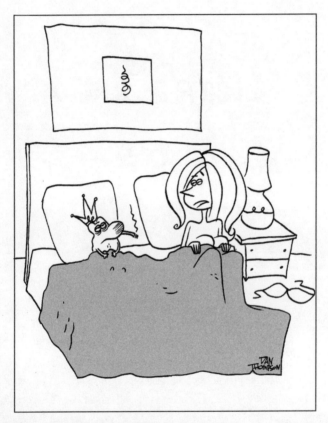

"Not exactly a Prince Charming in the sack, either."

Seventeen

Of Pillows and Scents:
Eroticize Your Love Den

To see, taste, touch, hear and smell the essence of a woman is to become a successful explorer; a modern Jacques Cousteau, a teacher and an A-plus student, all at the same time.

—DYLAN EDWARDS

You might be tempted to skip this chapter, thinking that what your abode looks like should have absolutely no bearing on your ability to seduce sexy women, but it does! As Pet of the Year Heather Vandeven put it, "I want a man, not a boy, so his bedroom better be put together." Remember, ambience is much more important to women than to men. If your place is dirty and unkempt, she will assume your body is too. As Pet Erica Ellyson put it, "Neatness is very important and no smells. The room should not look like he just had sex with someone else." Her sentiments are echoed by Pet of the Year Julie Strain, who says that "his bedroom should be clean and modern, but not the bachelor's sex pad with a strip pole. And don't let me see you turn the camera on!"

Women are also much more easily distractable than men, and little details like dust bunnies and pestulent pets could quickly get those Penthouse Pets that you worked so hard to bed out of your bedroom. So keep your place as clean as you possibly can, taking out garbage, washing floors, and dusting it on the day you invite her over. Make sure your clothes are hung up or stuffed in your drawers and that there are no odors. In addition, try to eliminate distracting stimuli from your bedroom, such as photos of your family, ex-girlfriends, or any other women (unless they are erotic works of art). Pet of the Month Brea Lynn emphasizes just that: "It is very important to me that I don't see pictures of him and ex-girlfriends or pictures of his parents."

Obviously, if you are only looking to have a one-night stand with a girl, you might not particularly care what she thinks of your place. However, if you are playing a long-term seduction strategy, then you should wait as long as possible to bring her to your place—remember, it is part of your mystique, and she should only be allowed in your space after she earns your trust. If at all possible, use her place or a hotel for the first couple of times that you hook up. When you do bring her to your place, make sure it is as clean and sexy as you can possibly make it.

Your place should be consistent with your prototype, otherwise you will be perceived as a phony impostor. I once dated a guy who came across as a suave, successful businessman. He dressed in impeccable suits, wore his alma mater ring, and acted accordingly, talking about his ventures and investments, taking me to nice restaurants, and paying for everything. I was impressed and turned on—until he invited me up to his apartment. His place was barely furnished, extremely messy, with dog poop conspicuously parked in the corner of the bathroom—and worst of all, he had a bitchy and nosy female roommate. Needless to say, my desire evaporated like the morning fog! Although he continued to act in a confident manner—he even lit up a Cuban cigar while offering me an expensive malt—his place blew away any pretense of his upscale attitude!

Similarly, if you want to come across as an intellectual, you better have some books by your night table. Pet Courtney Taylor, who is attracted to an intellectual prototype, prefers "a good, old-fashioned, neat bedroom, filled with intellectual books."

So the first thing you need to do is to make sure your bedroom doesn't scream for an extreme makeover. If you have a pest problem, make sure you become very friendly with your local exterminator. Then make sure your place is clean and organized. If your idea of cleaning is blowing the dust off your shelves, you need to hire a cleaning company. Sure, it'll cost you a couple hundred bucks a month, but the payoff is worth it. Last thing you want is your hottie turning into a wheezing, sniffling, and sneezing mess from all the dust must that reigns supreme under your bed.

So, if you want to make sure she does not bolt out of your bedroom, you should make sure your place is clean and your bathroom is well scrubbed, with lots of fresh cotton towels. However, if you really want to impress sexy women, you need to go a lot further—you need to create a hypnotic effect which speaks the sensory language of pleasure. Learn from Franz Mesmer, the eighteenth-century charlatan and founder of hypnotherapy, who "mesmerized" his patients with mystical music, exotic incense, stained glass, and mirrors. If you can afford to splurge on the upscale accessories, such as expensive sheets or goose-down pillows, do it. "Luxury—the sense that money has been spent or even wasted—adds to the feeling that the real world of duty and morality has been banished. Call it the brothel effect."[59] So turn your bedroom into a special oasis, a sanctuary, a place she will be coming to (and in) again and again. Here are some ways you can transform your pad into a cozy nest for all of your lovebirds:

Choose the Right Lighting

Nobody looks good under fluorescent lighting, and women particularly detest it. Try to get softer, warmer lighting, and make sure to install dimmer switches. Better yet, rely mainly on candlelight—you can even achieve the candlelight look without the danger of fire by purchasing fake candles. The softer the lighting, the more in the mood for sex she'll be, and the less likely she is to worry about the appearance of the cellulite on her thighs. As Playmate Charlotte Kemp put it: "I like soft, soft, soft—lights, sheets, music, candles."

Pick the Right Scents

Research has conclusively shown that scents have an impact on our moods. In one study, anxiety of patients undergoing an MRI was observed. When patients were submerged in a vanilla-like scent, 63 percent showed a reduction in anxiety. In another study, it was found that spiced apple and powder-fresh scents improved performance on a high-stress task.

An Austrian study focused on the effects of a citrus or orange scent in the waiting room of a dental office.[60] While patients were waiting for treatment, they were immersed in an orange smell. It was found that the odor had a relaxing effect, mostly on women. A lower level of anxiety, a more positive mood, and a greater sense of calmness were discovered to be direct effects of the orange odor. Take advantage of this odorific association, and make sure your place smells nice by ventilating it from time to time, hanging some air fresheners, adding potpourri, and/or getting some scented candles. But don't mix too many scents, and don't overdo it—combinations of strong smells trigger headaches in many women.

Scents to choose for your bedroom:

Chocolate	Vanilla	Orange	Cucumber
Strawberry	Musk	Jasmine	Peppermint
Patchouli	Ylang ylang		

Put Up Some Mirrors

Mirrors are a universal turn-on, so make sure your bedroom has at least a few. You can get a dresser with a mirror or mirrored closet doors. You are not the only one who will be enjoying the view—she, too, will get turned on if you begin feeling her up and undressing her in front of the mirror. You don't have to go as far as installing a mirror on the ceiling, though—that may scare away some of the more self-conscious hotties, who will immediately suspect that you might be a player.

Get Some Sexy Sheets

You might be perfectly fine with your old polyester sheets, but if you are going to be rolling on them with your honey bunnies, you'd better upgrade. Sheets that are satin, silk, or Egyptian cotton will feel much better against her bare naked flesh and will help create that special slippery action. When searching for the perfect bedding, think romance, sexiness, warmth, and comfort. You might want to choose bedding in darker, richer colors such as red, navy, or brown, which will conceal stains easier. Before she comes over, you can spray some of your pheromone-laden cologne on the sheets to evoke your scent and to make your bedding even more intimate. If you want to go a step further, you can get Sheets Gone Wild, which are illustrated with various sexual positions and come with a manual of sexual games (but keep them for when you begin seeing her on a regular basis—they might be too distracting for the first time you make love to her).

Invest in a Good Mattress

The last thing you want is a noisy, creaky, squeaky, shaky mattress when you are making love to the woman of your dreams. As Pet Brea Lynn emphasized, "The bed should be clean and made with a nice mattress, preferably one that doesn't squeak." And the last thing she expects to be popping up is an old spring in her behind when she springs in your bed. Whatever you do, though, stay away from a waterbed—the water movement is more distracting than erotic during lovemaking.

Stock Up on Pillows

You might be perfectly happy with the one pillow you've got, but she will find your bed far cozier if you add a few more—and you won't have to give yours up if she decides to stay over. Buy a couple of soft goose down pillows of different firmness and sizes. They will make convenient props for trying various sexual positions and for propping her hips up to maximize G-spot penetration (which you will read about below). If you have money to spend, invest in some love furniture from the Liberator (the wedge is a must-have for the right G-spot angle).

Hang Heavy, Thick Drapes

One of the most important concerns about a guy's pad expressed by centerfolds I interviewed was a sense of privacy. Make sure she will feel comfortable undressing in your bedroom, without fears of nosey neighbors or any other potential voyeurs intruding upon your sexual activities. Pet of the Year Julie Strain stresses the importance of the feeling of safety when it comes to a guy's bedroom. "I remember the time in high school when I was making out with a guy, I look up and there are five of his friends peering through the window," she jokes. Having blinds on the window provides basic protection from light and unwelcome eyes, while getting heavy, thick drapes guarantees the privacy with added coziness and romance.

Hang Some Classy Erotic Artwork

To reinforce the aura of erotica, hang some classy erotic art on your walls. To stay on the safe side, choose replicas of the masters, such as Ruben's nude, or originals of the modern pinup artists, such as Vargas prints. Make sure the artwork suits your prototype—being a modern girl I personally prefer replicas of surrealist painters such as Dali and Chagall, but if you want to come across as an old-fashioned romantic, hang a replica of *Birth of Venus*.

Install a Music Player

Make sure you have some way of playing music, whether it is a CD player, a radio, or an iPod with speakers. Have a few different types of music on hand: classical, rock, soft jazz, pop, and new age, to satisfy the taste of any hottie you bring. Music stimulates the release of endorphins, or feel-good hormones, in the brain. In addition, loud noise stimulates the sacculus, a small organ forming part of the balance-regulating vestibular system in our inner ear. The vestibular system has a connection to the hypothalamus, the part of the brain responsible for drives like hunger, sex, and hedonistic responses. That is why many people get a particularly pleasurable sensation when they listen to loud music. This high may mimic the thrills people get from swings and bungee jumping, where motion stimulates this balance center. To get the greatest high, make sure to turn the music volume up—the pleasure-inducing sacculus only appears to be sensitive to loud noises—above 90 decibels (having said that, avoid blaring the music, or you'll have to wear a hearing aid when you get older). If you hit a CD super-sale, get a few identical mood CDs—this way you can give her one as a gift to remind her of the great evening you had together (remember the positive associations rule?).

Put Out Some Fresh Flowers

Finally, if you want to add a winning touch of sensuality and romance, buy some fresh flowers. Go for unusual or wildflowers instead of the typical ones, like carnations. Stay away from roses because the scent of roses has been shown to actually inhibit sexual desire. Of course, if you have a green thumb, it's good to have a few plants around, but don't keep the wilted ones.

Have Drinks and Snacks Handy

Always have some alcohol handy—not to get her sloshed but to offer her a classy drink. Hot women love champagne, so invest in an expensive bottle. Wines and liquors are also good to keep around. Most women love chocolate, so always have some handy. Ice cream is also a woman's favorite snack (make it a fat-free one, to minimize her guilt).

Sex Aids

Always have protection measures and some lubricant around, but make sure they are safely out of sight until you need them. Never, ever offer a woman a used sex toy. You can offer her the one that is still in the wrapper, but I would wait until you've been with that hottie a few times before turning to a vibrator for additional excitement.

Clean and Comfy Bathroom

Women spend a lot of time in the bathroom—shaving, doing their hair, and fixing their makeup, so bathrooms are particularly important to them. Make sure yours is clean and you have an extra razor and toothbrush handy. Big fluffy terry towels and soft robes are also a plus!

Working Thermostat

Although this seems self-explanatory, I feel I have to stress the importance of the optimal temperature because of a few experiences I've had. One time I had sex at a guy's house and his AC system was down (because he hadn't paid his electric bill) and we were both absolutely soaked in sweat. Needless to say, this was not a pleasant experience. Similarly, if your heat is not working, she is unlikely to want to get naked.

Doing most of the above will guarantee that she will enjoy the time she spends in your love den. But what about a television set, you may ask? Believe it or not, not having a TV will not break the deal for her. While having a TV set can be helpful once you want to get into mutual sexual fantasy exploration, you can easily explore her fantasies in other ways. As you will learn below, women respond better to aural fantasies than they do to visual ones, and romance novels will provide a far faster way of turning her on than the XXX-rated fare.

TIP #21: Turn your place into a love den by keeping it clean and organized. If you want her to love every minute she spends at your place and look forward to coming back, choose the right lighting, put up some mirrors, pick the right scents, get some sexy sheets, invest in a good mattress, stock up on pillows, hang heavy, thick drapes, hang some classy erotic artwork, install a music player, and put out some fresh flowers. ✦

Eighteen

Beyond Buttocks and Breasts:
Being a Smooth Operator

I want a man with a slow hand . . .

— THE POINTER SISTERS, "Slow Hand"

Believe it or not, a lot of hot women—including, very likely, your favorite centerfold—don't know the difference between a great lover and a lousy one. If their experience has been with hot-looking men or "players," those guys are often so into themselves and their own narcissistic pleasure that they don't know how to, or don't care to, give pleasure to their partners. If the hotties have spent their time in bed with older, wealthy men, they have had to deal with ED (erectile dysfunction) and lack of staying power. Indeed, even with the average Joes they may have had sex with, their very beauty and sex appeal is likely to have been their downfall when it came to their own sexual satisfaction: guys get so turned on and eager when it comes to sex with a hottie that they often rush it and can't last more than the proverbial "two minutes and out"!

In my own case, it was many years after I became sexually active—and many lovers in and out of my bed—that I even had an orgasm during sex; and even now, I would rate only about 10 percent of the men I've been with as being even "good" in bed. The rest ranged from "mediocre" to just plain lousy; and I'm not the only centerfold with that experience. Just about every hot model I've talked to has had similar complaints—and believe me, we *always* talk about men when we're together! For a time, I believed that having bad, or at least unsatisfying, sexual experiences just "came with the territory" of being a glamorous woman.

I'm telling you this because getting your dream girl into bed is likely to be the opportunity of a lifetime to totally impress her with your lovemaking prowess, to turn yourself from just an average guy who she likes well enough to sleep with into a superhero in her eyes. If she has never experienced "super-sex"—that mind-blowing, multiple-orgasmic, breathtaking sexual experience that the romance novels all talk about, but which few women experience—then you have the chance to be "the One" who initiates her into the rarified company of truly satisfied women; and if you accomplish that, you can just about write your own ticket for repeat visits of her eager, naked body to your bed. And if you are looking for a relationship beyond the bedroom, you can be sure that the flood of endorphins and oxytocin that super-sex brings with it will have a profound influence on her mind's ability to perceive you as her true Prince Charming.

Of course, you are now asking: what superhuman, acrobatic, impossibly pretzel-twisting performance do I have to produce in order to get her to think I am such a fabulous lover? The answer is "none of the above." Any perfectly average guy, with just average strength and no particular athletic skills, can be the greatest lover a supermodel has ever known. As we will see, it doesn't take a fantastic body, or a big penis, or male-model good looks to turn yourself into the hero of her dreams in the intimate game of lovemaking. It only takes a few simple skills or qualities:

a) **Patience**—taking the time to get her fully aroused *before* initiating direct clitoral (for oral sex) or vaginal (for intercourse) stimulation and continuously checking for her feedback;

b) **Thoroughness**—stimulating as many of her erotic zones as possible, so that her entire body is aroused and building sexual tension;

c) **Dedication**—believing that your goal is to maximize her pleasure and to give her as many orgasms as she is capable of experiencing—even ahead of your own satisfaction—and convincing her that you mean it, so she learns to expect such pleasure from you;

d) **Delaying ejaculation**—holding off your own orgasm during intercourse until she has experienced one (or more) orgasms, is close to coming, or is at least enjoying herself; and

e) **Creating a romantic aura**—getting her to believe throughout the sexual encounter that you are interested in more than conquering her body, but, instead, that you care about her as a person.

That's it! Master those five skills, and you will have even the hottest women you have ever fantasized about wanting you again and again. Believe me. Even writing down these five qualities makes me pine for the man that can fulfill them! Indeed, I expect that I will have to change my panties numerous times while writing this chapter, as the kind of man that can achieve all five of these criteria is so rare in my experience that just writing about them sets off intense sexual fantasies in my mind. So, if you want to be part of my fantasies, or those of other hot women you are dreaming about, pay careful attention to the sections that follow. They may literally change your life!

TIP #22: Every hot woman dreams of incredible sex, and very few women actually get to experience it. You can be the man that no woman ever forgets and against whom she measures all of her subsequent lovers if you take the time to fully and thoroughly stimulate her body, do it with dedication, delay your orgasm until she has hers, and create an aura of romance while doing all of the above. ✦

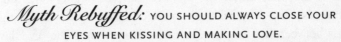

Myth Rebuffed: YOU SHOULD ALWAYS CLOSE YOUR EYES WHEN KISSING AND MAKING LOVE.

Most men and women close their eyes when making out and having sex. To achieve better sex through greater intimacy, renowned psychologist David Schnarch recommends "eyes-open sex" in his book *The Passionate Marriage.* According to Dr. Schnarch, only about 30 percent of all couples have sex with their eyes open, and less than half of these can have "eyes-open orgasms." Most people have to tune out their partner in order to have an orgasm. Dr. Schnarch advises having sex with your eyes open, as well as having enough light in the room in order to see each other. But "seeing" doesn't mean looking at each other's bodies—it involves letting your partner look into your eyes and your soul. This practice of intense eye contact is known as "soul-gazing" in Tantric teaching, and it is supposed to transmit sexual energy. So, the next time you are kissing and having sex with your hottie, do not turn off the lights and do not close your eyes. Keep your eyes open throughout the encounter and gaze steadily into her eyes, even if she does not reciprocate the whole time. *At the moment of orgasm, look into her eyes*—she will be electrified by the connection you experience!

How to Prolong Foreplay as Much as Possible

*Seems to me the basic conflict between men and women, sexually,
is that men are like firemen. To men, sex is an emergency, and
no matter what we're doing we can be ready in two minutes.
Women, on the other hand, are like fire. They're very exciting,
but the conditions have to be exactly right for it to occur.*

—Jerry Seinfeld

The number one complaint that just about all women have about
men is that they almost never have the patience to wait until a
woman is turned on all the way before wanting to plunge their
penis between her love lips, or even before wanting to dive down
for an attack on her clit. Thus, a man of real patience is a woman's
dream; and extended foreplay may not be the shortest, but it is by
far the best, route to her love nest.

Start Early and Make It Often

Foreplay doesn't start when you are naked and in bed. Any lesbian
will tell you that a good sexual experience for a woman begins any-
time, whenever the thought of sex strikes the two of you. It may be
a word, a glance, or the sure knowledge that since you are already
lovers, one or both of you will want to initiate sex that night. If that
is you, start your foreplay long before bedtime. To build up her
anticipation and to stimulate her arousal, try sensuously touching
her body from time to time during the day, or holding her hands
and gently stroking or massaging her fingers. Look her squarely in
the eyes and smile, with one of those "knowing" smiles that says
you are thinking of the pleasure you will bring her. Stimulate her
thoughts of sex with words and hints at what you would like to do
with her come bedtime. Use every opportunity—a movie or TV
show you watch together, a news item you read or see, or a passage
from the book you are reading—as an excuse to casually mention

something about sex and sexual pleasure. Never press the issue, or prolong your touches or kisses, or act needy. Just give her continual but short reminders of your interest in and desire for her, and let her mind dwell on them. It will!

Make "Getting Ready" Part of the Foreplay

Some guys, when it comes to bedtime and sex is on their minds, just strip down to the buff, hop into bed, and start stroking themselves, waiting for their woman to do likewise. What a crock! Unless they are already overcome with lust, most women would find that kind of "let's strip and do it" behavior a real downer. Beautiful women always need to take time to get ready for bed. The ideal lover will use this time as part of his foreplay. While she moisturizes her face, brush her hair for her, using long, sensuous strokes with gentle smoothing with your hands, letting them trail down her neck and back. Tell her what you think of her skin, eyes, and hair as you watch her in her makeup mirror, with a little graphic detail of what you are going to do to enjoy those aspects of her face and body when she is finished.

Whenever possible, be the one that undresses her—you can tell her that is one of your most favorite acts of foreplay, so you can make it a habit—and make that undressing a sensual experience. Slow unbuttoning and removal of each article; gentle, undemanding and skin-smoothing caresses; and the look in your eyes that you are enjoying every inch of her body that is being revealed will get her shivering with anticipation. If she wants, let her do the same to you. Her fingers on your body will stimulate her at the same time. Just keep your excitement totally under control—your role as "great lover" means you are going to put her pleasure first, so you have to hold back your own.

Set the Tone for Long Foreplay

When she is finished with her nighttime preparations and/or undressed, and you lead her or guide her to your side of the bed, you should let her know, either directly in words or by your actions, that you intend to give her a long, sensuous foreplay session. When a man tells me he intends to kiss and/or caress every inch of my body, lingering at every erotic area, I get aroused just hearing those words. And when I know from experience that he is both capable and willing to do just that, I start lubricating at his first touch. Most women respond in just that way. It's what we dream of in our erotic fantasies—seemingly "endless" foreplay until we are wound up tighter than a mummy with sexual tension and ready to simply explode with pleasure—so when a man promises such an experience and can deliver on it, it is a huge turn-on.

Remember: the more you get her thinking about and imagining the upcoming orgasms and sexual pleasure, the hotter she will get. Women are aroused as much by mental and emotional imagery as by purely visual and tactile stimuli; so your "fucking in her mind" is all part of good foreplay.

Soften Your Touch

When you begin touching her, make sure to start with the softest imaginable touch. The softer the touch, the more aroused she will become. You can even try an erotic form of tickling, called *pattes d'arraignée,* or, literally translated from French, "spider's legs." It is done by using the tips of the fingers for the lightest possible touch, aiming to touch not the skin but the tiny skin hairs, not on the genitals but on other sensitive areas such as the chest, belly, insides of arms and thighs, armpits, and the back. The idea is that the extreme lightness of the touch is electric and erotic, like a light breeze brushing over the skin. When you see goose bumps on her skin, or when she starts to moan, slowly increase the pressure of your touch.

Keep Away from Her Pussy

Finally, when you do get to the touchy-feely-kissy part of foreplay, don't touch her genitals! I repeat. Do not touch her genitals—at least not until after you have already gotten her very aroused. This is entirely counterintuitive for men, who love nothing more than beginning foreplay by having their women grab their willies and start sucking on them vigorously. But women are different—like I had to tell you that, right? A woman's genitals are more sensitive to rough handling; until her clitoris, vaginal lips, and vaginal walls are fully lubricated and engorged with blood, she is likely to feel your finger, lip, or tongue strokes as rough, certainly not very pleasurable. Thus, good foreplay means great patience in addressing all the other erogenous zones on her body, getting her fully aroused and wet *before* addressing her genitals.

How long do you wait? The average woman requires anywhere from 20 to 45 minutes to become fully aroused from a "standing start." All depends on the woman, her level of sexual need and hormonal flow, her time of the month,[61] and a host of other factors. You need to learn the signs of her arousal—the sounds she makes, the way she squirms or writhes, the level of sexual flush showing in her cheeks, the tightness or stiffness of her thighs and belly, her responsive caresses on your body, the passion in her kisses—to judge when she is ready for direct genital stimulation, and then for tongue, finger, or penile penetration. Thus, patience is especially important during your initial lovemaking sessions with a woman, so you can observe and learn those clues to her arousal. After you have watched her go from a resting state to full arousal and then orgasm a few dozen times, you should have a pretty good idea of when to step up the action.

TIP #23: Prolong your foreplay as much as possible by touching her as often as you can and as softly as you can, setting the tone for a long foreplay and keeping your hands away from her genitals for as long as possible. ✦

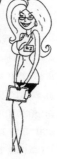

The Clit to Lip Connection

Besides being the experts on extending female orgasms, Drs. Vera and Steve Bodansky have a couple of other tricks up their sleeves. In their book *To Bed or Not to Bed,* they describe an exercise that teaches you to connect your hottie's erogenous zones to her genitals, so that stimulation of those erogenous zones leads to a pleasant stirring in her pants. The easiest thing to connect is her clit to her mouth. According to the instructions, start to masturbate her lubricated clitoris until it becomes engorged. Then place some lubricant on your other hand and start stroking the lips of her mouth while continuing to rub her clitoris, trying to keep both strokes similar to each other in pressure, length of stroke, and speed. After stroking both areas simultaneously for a while, remove your hand from her lips for a few seconds, while continuing to stroke her clitoris; then alternate; then return to rubbing both areas at the same time. It sounds a bit kinky, but it works! After a couple of weeks of this rather enjoyable practice, her clit should awaken the minute you begin kissing or rubbing her lips!

HOW TO BE THOROUGHLY SENSUAL

Don't stint on foreplay, be inventive.
                    —DR. RUTH WESTHEIMER

As part of the extended foreplay that you want to provide your dream girl—assuming you want her to think of you as her super lover—you should apply the second rule: thoroughly stimulate every part of her body. Why? First, because you need to take the time to get her fully aroused before you can hop on and bang away, and it's boring to spend all that time on one thing. Second, variety is not only the "spice of life" but it is also a critical component of great sex, so the more varied your foreplay is each time, the more exciting it is. To attain that variety, you need to learn every possible area of her body and all the different ways to stimulate them.

Her Top 12 Underused Moan Zones

1. Rub her wrists. This seemingly innocuous zone is a great place to start your foreplay. The inside of an arm is a very sensitive zone due to thinner skin, and it is responsive to light stimulation. Begin by taking her hand and rubbing her fingers, then slowly proceed to her inner wrist zone, gently brushing the tips of your fingers all the way up to the inner elbow area, then up to the underarm. The back of your hand can "accidentally" brush against her breast, but do not make it obvious.

2. Excite her eyes. The area above and on her eyelid has a great concentration of nerve endings; the area between the outer corner of the eye and the cheekbone is also very sensitive. In short, after giving her mouth some nice passionate kisses, you should pay equal attention to the rest of her face!

3. Cherish her cheeks and chin. The cheeks and chin are remarkably sensitive zones. Infants respond to cheek stimulation by turning their heads and opening their mouths (the so-called rooting reflex). As adults we continue to enjoy gentle cheek stimulation. Gently brush the back of your hand against her cheek, and then touch or trace her lips. Then stroke her chin with your fingers, gently gripping it and drawing it to you for a soft kiss.

4. Give her an ear-gasm. Most women are extremely sensitive behind and over their earlobes. Alas, few men have the "ear fetish." Surprise her with some hot nibbling, licking, and kissing her behind and on her ears and you'll be hearing her moan in your ear!

5. Stroke her shoulders. Believe it or not, the areas from the back and sides of the neck to the ends of the shoulder blades are the most erotic zones on a woman's body. Some women can even come from neck-to-shoulder stimulation! Massage, kisses, even love bites are OK here. Why do you think Count Dracula always snared the hot chicks?

6. Nuzzle her navel. All women like to be stroked and kissed from the rib cage down to the top of her pubic V; the closer you come to her pubes, the hotter she will feel. But this is a prime "tease" zone. Hold off on grabbing those genitals, but make her think you will. Every time you get close, move your lips or hands back toward her navel until she is simply dying to have you clamp down on her clit.

7. Go treasure hunting. The aptly named "Treasure Trail" is the most sensitive area of a woman's lower torso. This is the crease or line that extends across a woman's lower abdomen from one hipbone to the other, passing right over the top of the region covered with pubic hair (in its unshaved state). It crisscrosses the navel-to-Z zone and should be stimulated teasingly until you get her squirming.

8. **Tease her tootsies.** This is the ultimate foreplay tease. Just when she thinks you will surely start in on her clit and vaginal area, you shift way down to her toes. Many women get turned on by toe-sucking and foot worship; but when you start in on those little piggies after doing zones 1–5, she can be driven mad with desire—especially if you take plenty of time working each toe, instep, heel, arch, etc.

9. **Knead behind her knees.** The skin behind the knees is thin and soft and very responsive to touch because the nerves are close to the surface. Stopping to attend to this zone as you kiss and fondle each leg from toes to crotch helps build up the suspense.

10. **Caress the crease.** One of the more erotic zones on a woman's body is the crease between the curve of her buttocks and the top of her thighs, known as the sacral crease. Stroking or running a finger along that crease usually produces a strong erotic response. Work on it while you play with her ass.

11. **Worship her booty.** The buttocks themselves are a strong erogenous zone, but they need to be approached slowly, after the other zones have been stimulated. But when you've got her really warmed up, anything goes, from squeezing to spanking.

12. **Tantalize her thighs.** This is the last area to be stimulated before moving to her genitals. Don't overlook it, though, as soft kisses and light fingertip stroking from her knees right up to (but not including) her vulva and clitoris will send her into that loud moaning state that proclaims her readiness for genital stimulation.

So, guys, if you want to put to rest all those "not enough fore-play" complaints and get a reputation as a maestro of the bedroom, give her the twelve-course meal above. You'll soon have her eating out of your hand—and likely eating the rest of you as well!

◆ ◆ ◆

Of course, you will want to spend considerable time on her breasts too. But you must stimulate her breasts in the right way to qualify for the title of super lover. Always start with gentle touches, cupping a full breast in a hand or kissing the tops of the breasts near the neck. Try to spiral your caresses from the outer edges of the breast inward toward the nipple. Bring a line of kisses from the sensitive areas of her neck slowly to her breast edges, and then work toward the nipple. The areola and the nipple are the most sensitive areas of the breast and should be the last areas to receive their tribute of kisses and caresses. *Starting off with just grabbing a nipple or squeezing a breast is a real turnoff for most women.* Only after working up to it slowly can you then knead or even lightly pinch the engorged nipples. *Some women feel that there is a "hotline" between their nipples and their clitoris,* so every time you stimulate their breasts there is a double effect.[62]

Now, do you use all of these techniques and attack every moan zone every time? Of course not! Treat this list as a playlist or "mix tape" of her favorite songs; choose a different concert for her each time you make love. As you get to know the things that turn her on the most (and the fastest), you will want to use those techniques more frequently, but variety is extremely important in keeping sex from getting stale and "routine," so if you want to keep her coming back for more, mix it up! Besides, you won't always have time for such a thorough lovemaking—a quickie can be a nice way to change up your sexual script from time to time.

Also, you can stimulate several areas on her body simultaneously. While your lips are on her face, your hands don't have to just sit there on her back. They should be roaming her body, caressing and touching every part they can reach. As they roam, they can lightly brush over her pubic mound, or your finger can swirl briefly through her pubic hair as a reminder of what is to come; but otherwise, they should stay away until she is ready for that part. You want to work her whole body into your foreplay so she builds sexual tension everywhere—and by the way, using your hands when kissing her is a great idea, even when you are fully clothed and merely greeting each other or saying good night. That way, she learns to associate every kiss with sexual arousal; and positive associations like that will keep your love life flaming.

Foreplay is not just all hands, lips, and skin. The aural senses are just as important as the tactile. One of my best Pet friends told me that she wasn't too impressed physically with a guy she was dating, but she found him a super lover in bed because he continually talked to her while he played with her body. From whispered compliments on each body part he was caressing, to statements as to what he was going to do to her next, to the moaning and squirming he expected from her when he shifted to a new technique, he never let her forget that she was being adored, sexually aroused, and being brought to orgasm. She said she simply couldn't help achieving climax when verbally stimulated in this way, no matter what his hands and lips might be doing. And then, whenever they were out on a date, he only had to whisper some of those same words in her ear, and she was instantly turned on and ready to end the date with some hot sex. Guess what? She married him, despite the fact that he was the least handsome boyfriend I'd ever seen her with. So never forget that sweet talking can land you a sweet thing!

Use words to cement your babe's fixation on you in other ways as well. Coming up with secret "pet" names for each other—or for key body parts on each other's bodies—is one way to build the intimacy that great lovers contemplate; and telling her in advance what delights you have planned for her in bed will raise her level of arousal long before you reach the bedroom. You can even build a "secret world" in bed, with different names for different sexual actions and activities that only the two of you know. Mixing a little mysticism into your love play not only adds to the romantic allure you are creating but it also makes you "special" in her eyes, because only you can live in this secret sexual world with her. If no other man can make her cum from the "Sumatran Swirl"—your secret name for her favorite form of oral sex—because they don't even know the name she associates with it, pretty soon you will be the main man in her sex life!

TIP #23: Impress her by discovering her hidden moan zones, such as her back, navel, or the delicate skin behind her knee. By making sex a full body experience you will impress her further than any of her previous lovers— because they were probably genitally focused, like most men. ✦

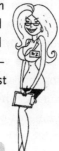

Eight Sure Ways to Make Her Really Hot and Bothered

1. Tantalize her aurally. While men are visual creatures, women get aroused by verbal stimulation. Describe to her what you will do to her sexually—in graphic and explicit detail—or tell her an erotic XXX-rated story involving her as the main character. A story that has her performing in her favorite sexual fantasy will have her playing with herself even before you touch her!

2. Take charge. Order her to prepare herself for having sex with you. Give her detailed instructions on how to prepare her body in the shower, put on your favorite perfume and lingerie, etc. Order her to masturbate in front of you, with or without a toy, until you see the sexual flush in her cheeks. Inspect every inch of her slowly and silently until she is squirming with anticipation. Do this right and your two-minute fuck will be enough to get her off too!

3. Shave her. Many women find that their genitals are more sensitive after being shaved. Take your time lathering her privates and shaving both her vaginal and anal orifices. Test each millimeter of her skin for smoothness with your fingers. Oil her afterwards. Call her "My Baby" and cradle her in your lap. She'll be dripping before you know it!

4. Feel her up. An erotic massage is a good heat builder. Start with very gentle touches known as *pattes d' arraignée,* or spider's legs, designed to touch just the hairs on her skin. Then slowly proceed to giving her firmer touches, leading to a deeper massage. It's prolonged foreplay, but it sounds like more fun when you call it a massage.

5. Extend your kissing. Kiss her not only on the mouth but also on the face, the back of her neck, behind her ears, on the ears, from her neck to her shoulders—everywhere you can reach above her breasts—until she pushes your head down south. Her push tells you her temperature is reaching the boiling point!

6. Get her moving. Ask her to model some lingerie, strip, dance, or pose for you. You can even take photos—or touch yourself while she strips. Putting on a show for you, and watching you get horny, will put her in a very sexy mood. You didn't think you could make out without touching? Well, think again!

7. Explore her body. Touch and caress every inch of her body, exploring unexpected erogenous zones, such as the backs of her knees, her armpits, or her toes. Or use her body as a dinner plate or snack dish, nibbling food or sipping wine from her curves. Each little slurp, lick, or bite will make her hungry for some steamy action!

8. Sharpen her senses. Dulling one of the senses is known to increase another, so blindfold her while caressing her all over, or put earphones on her while moving a buzzing vibrator around her erotic zones. Less can be more when it comes to sensual play!

Nineteen

The Clitoris and G-Spot: Making Her Come First

In the case of some women, orgasms take quite a bit of time. Before signing on with such a partner make sure you are willing to lay aside, say, the month of June, with sandwiches having to be brought in. —BRUCE JAY FRIEDMAN

The third quality that differentiates a super lover from the average-to-awful clods with whom most beautiful women are stuck is a willingness to put *her* pleasure first. For men, having sex almost invariably means having an orgasm. Not so with women. Many women do not experience an orgasm from the average male's coital efforts; and even among those who do, they may achieve orgasm only 50 percent or even as little as 25 percent of the time. One-third of all women—including a like percentage of your favorite hotties—rarely reach orgasm at all from vaginal sex. Naturally enough, these women are not particularly impressed by the sexual skills of the men they bed; and many of them fall into the habit of faking orgasms in order not to disappoint their partners, or out of fear of displeasing them.

This doesn't have to be the case, though. Almost all women can achieve orgasm through clitoral stimulation, either by masturbation or oral sex; and even women who have difficulty reaching orgasm from intercourse will be able to experience a climax if it is preceded by clitoral stimulation to near-orgasm (or to an initial orgasm plus further stimulation). Therefore, any man who wants to can virtually "guarantee" that his dream girl will enjoy a great orgasm every time she jumps in his bed, simply by deciding in advance that he will not stop his foreplay and begin intercourse until he has brought her to orgasm from oral or manual stimulation.

In addition, putting her orgasm first every time will increase your romantic stature in her eyes. Even if you aren't interested in a committed relationship, this is a big plus, as female sexual desire is always linked, consciously or subconciously, with romance. So the more she thinks you care for her, and that you want more than to merely use her body for your own pleasure, the more she will desire you and the more eager she will be to accept your invitations to repeat performances in your bed. There is nothing better you can do to inculcate this feeling in your dream girl than telling her and showing her that you put her pleasure before your own. Such an attitude is so rare in the men most hotties sleep with that it ensures that you will aways be special in her eyes.

For these reasons, some leading "sexologists," like Ian Kerner, author of *She Comes First: The Thinking Man's Guide to Pleasuring a Woman,* argue that men should adopt the rule that a man should always withhold his own climax until his partner has achieved hers, using oral sex as the best means to achieve this goal. While I don't agree that there are any "rules" that should be rigidly applied to sex, as variety and surprise are the "spice" that makes sex fun, the principle of "she comes first" is one I believe most men should strive to meet if they want to score well and often with a woman.

TIP #24: Make sure she always comes first. Period. ✦

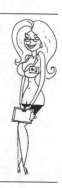

How to Make Love to Her Sweet Spot:
The Art of Oral Pleasuring

Some men love oral sex . . . If you find a man like this, treat him well. Feed him caviar and don't let your girlfriends catch a glimpse of him.
                                    —Cynthia Heimel

Never do with your hands what you could do better with your mouth.
                                    —Cherry Vanilla

Up to now, I have focused on the foreplay needed to fully arouse a woman and the reasons why you should want to bring her to a clitoral orgasm every time you bed her. Now let's address my favorite subject: how to give good head to a hottie. It's my favorite subject, since I am one of those women who climax much more easily from clitoral stimulation. A man who would be my lover has to be good at oral sex. A weak tongue or fumbly fingers just won't cut it! About half of the centerfolds I know or have interviewed for this book agree that great oral sex skills are either number one or number two on the list of desired attributes they look for in a sex partner. So, you should not consider mastering the art of oral pleasuring to be an "extra" in your arsenal of sexual techniques; it will be the foundation stone on which your overall sexual prowess—and thus your desirability as a lover for your dream girl—will be judged.

Start Softly, and Work Up to Heavier Stimulation

The key to cunnilingus, or giving good head to a woman, is to start softly and gradually increase pressure and speed until she is on her way to an orgasmic summit; and then hold that pressure, tempo, and technique until she hits her peak. Most men make the mistake when they go down on a woman of initiating an immediate mouth-mashing, heavy sucking, or licking attack on her poor little love button—or worse, they try to drive their tongue deep in her vagina. That kind of overeager, ignorant approach is more likely to destroy all the sexual tension she has built up from your careful, prolonged foreplay. Forget all those porn DVDs you might have seen. That's not the way a woman really wants to be stimulated in this sensitive area.

Instead, when your foreplay has gotten her sufficiently aroused, wet your fingers in her fluids (or you can use your saliva—or hers, as having her suck your fingers is incredibly sexy) and rub gentle circles around and over her vaginal lips. Then spread your first two fingers and lightly rub the V of your spread fingers along both sides of her clitoral sheath. Close the V just enough to cause the clitoral hood to pull back, revealing her clit. Repeat these steps a few times; then, with the clitoral hood pulled back, kiss her clitoris, softly, lovingly, and wetly. This is good to set the mood as one of romance and appreciation for her femininity; and it is a reminder of the pleasures to come. Soft kisses all over her vaginal area strengthen that mood. Make sure that you wet your lips before each kiss or mouth-to-genital touch (and that your fingernails are trimmed and smooth before even starting this process)!

You can follow up these first kisses by lightly licking all around her clit, then over the top of the hood. Pulling back the hood and using mainly the tip of your tongue, flick your tongue back and forth and up and down over the exposed clit. See if you can make it swell and stand up like a miniature penis. After a light and gentle beginning, you can step up the oral action by lapping at her clitoris with full tongue strokes, like a cat laps up cream. As always, start slowly and gradually increase the tempo, always using a rhythmic pace. You can also expand the lapping to include her vaginal lips within each stroke; or, use a wet finger to stroke and tease those lips while your tongue is focused on her clit.

Add variety to your pleasuring by closing your lips over her clit (using just your lips, not your teeth) and pulling back, letting the clit slide out of your mouth—or push it out with your tongue. Then add a gentle sucking on the clit as an alternative. You can include her whole vulva in your mouth for a time, as women love being "deep mouthed." Another technique is to take her clit firmly between your lips and hum. That will cause your lips to vibrate, giving her clit the sensation she might remember from using her favorite sex toy.

"Steady As She Goes . . ."

Most women climax more easily with repetitive and continuous stimulation, rather than from harsher or widely varying tongue or finger action. So use her moans and squirms as clues to maintain the rhythm and pressure that produced those responses. If you get tired, switch from your tongue to your moistened fingers, rubbing them back and forth over her clit in a window-wiper motion. When her clit is already engorged, you can also pinch it, tap it, and even lightly spank it to add to her arousal. Then return to your oral pleasuring. Since it may take anywhere from 3 to 30 minutes to bring her to orgasm, depending on her state of readiness before you start going down on her, be relaxed and patient and enjoy the sights, sounds, and smells that evidence her pleasure with your efforts. Eventually, though, you will hear her breathing grow very quick, feel her belly and/or thighs grow taut with tension, or note other signs of her impending orgasm.

Tightening the Spring until It's Sprung

At that point, you have several choices. If you want to build her sexual tension higher to produce a more intense and powerful orgasm, you should "back off," stimulating the areas around and on the sides of the clit and vaginal lips but not touching the clit itself until she cools off somewhat. Then resume doing what you were doing until you sense her approaching climax once again. You can repeat this approach-and-pull-back technique several times, until she is near frenzied in her need for release.

If you want her to climax with your penis inside her, you can bring her close to orgasm and then kiss your way up her body until you can penetrate her fully and begin intercourse. Do you want your girl to be begging and pleading for you to impale her? Torturing her with several near-orgasms from your tongue and fingers is one good way to get there. Finally, if you want to bring her off orally first, you just bring her to (or back to) that "peak" of near orgasm with the technique that seemed to get the biggest response and continue doing it until she goes "over the top" and into orgasm. Don't make the mistake of trying to lick harder or faster—it's the rhythmic, repetitive, continuous action that counts. *And don't stop the action unless she tells you to.* She wants the same stimulation that brought her to the brink to continue, unchanged and unabated, all the way through her orgasm, which may last for up to a minute if it's a "Big O." And if you do pull off the "Big O," you are more than halfway home to becoming a super lover in her mind.

That's all there is to it: (1) start gently and work up to harder pressure and faster strokes; (2) find the rhythm and technique that get her moaning and squirming, and take her to the brink with them; and (3) when you have her where you want her, go for the "Big O" by continuing your steady, unrelenting clit action in her favorite mode. Shame on you guys who think it's hard to give good head. It's so easy a caveman could do it—and they probably did!

TIP # 25: When pleasuring her orally, always start softly and work up to heavier stimulation, paying careful attention to her responses, building up and then backing off until she grabs your head and keeps it there—at that point, don't stop the action unless she tells you to. ✦

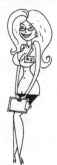

How to Catch that Elusive "Venus Butterfly"

A lot of men who are trying to be really "super" in the oral sex department want to know how to perform the "Venus Butterfly," that mystical, secret oral technique that had all the female lawyers going crazy on the TV show *L.A. Law* a few years ago. However, there is no such technique described in the annals of sexology, so I suspect that the writers of the TV show simply made up the name and, of course, never revealed the "secret." But the effects described by those breathless legal beagles on *L.A. Law* can be achieved by combining a clitoral orgasm with a G-spot orgasm. That "double O" is sure to get her shuddering in pure delight; and while it is hard to pull off, she will always appreciate the effort. There are two well-known ways to go for the "double":

The first is a combination of the window-wiper clitoral stimulation with the "come hither" method of G-spot stimulation. The G-spot, as you all know—or should know—is the raised and slightly ridged area of her vagina which is located on the upper (front) side of her love canal about one inch in from her vaginal opening. It is best found with a crooked finger wiggled in a "come hither" motion. When your fingertip encounters a slightly rough or ridged patch, that is the "G"; touching it will often produce a gasp or noticeable reaction. Once you have zeroed in on her G-spot, you can best stimulate it with either a tapping motion or a "come hither" stroking. When you combine G-spot stimulation with the oral techniques described above you are doubling her pleasure; and if you can balance the two types of pleasuring, you can give her a twin climax from both her clitoris and her G-spot at the same time. To make it work, you should bring her close to climax several times with clitoral stimulation, each time backing off to increase the amount of sexual tension in her body and raising her clit's sensitivity to the maximum. When you feel that she is about to climax from tapping or stroking a finger on her "G," you should then add some quick, firm, two-finger "window wiping" on her clit. Time it right and she will experience both orgasms simultaneously.

The other method involves putting your hands together, inserting the index and middle fingers of both hands into her vagina where they massage her G-spot, while using your two thumbs to stimulate her clitoris, with a back-and-forth motion. If you can use your last two fingers to stimulate her anus or her perineum (the area between her anus and vagina), so much the better. When you coordinate these motions, the movements of your hands resemble the flapping of butterfly wings, which may have been the idea behind the "Venus Butterfly." You should approach her nirvana moment the same way as in the first method, bringing her close and backing off until her clitoris is ready to trigger an explosion, then concentrating on her G-spot until she is ready to come from that stimulation as well. Whichever method you use, that "double O" is pure heaven for a woman! (Pardon me, but I need a panty change just describing this.)

The Taste of Love

Some guys have trouble performing oral sex on a woman because they don't like the taste of her vaginal fluids. While she should make sure her genitals are clean before you start—and showering or bathing together is a great way to add to your foreplay—you can also negate any unwanted odors lingering in her love nest by using fla-voring. Everything from chocolate to spicy condiments can be used to turn her pubic area into your favorite eating establishment. Hav-ing a menthol cough drop in your mouth while sucking on her clit is especially arousing to her, as it imparts a bite of coolness to your suction and can produce a tingling sensation in her clit. Others use ice in their mouths to produce an even colder sensation, or hot pep-per sauce on their lips to add some burning sensation to the fire in their lapping. An even bigger smorgasbord of flavors is available to make oral pleasuring tasty, with honey, various fruit syrups, whipped cream, and chocolate being the most popular. Just be sure to keep the sugary concoctions and the ice on the outside of her vulva and her clitoris, and not let them get inside her vagina itself, where they may cause yeast infections or damage delicate tissues.

Even if your honey's honeypot smells and tastes delicious with-out sauces and spices, using flavorings in your oral pleasuring is a good way to create variety and keep her interested in your love-making. When you show up at your bedside with a can of whipped cream in hand, she will have a good idea that the white stuff will soon be decorating her muff. Just the thought might start her lubricating. Savoring each little morsel of the flavorful ingredients you use will help you prolong your foreplay and your oral pleasur-ing, leading her to experience more intense oral "O's." After all, they don't call oral sex "eating out" for nothing! Bon appétit.

TIP #26: If you want to give her even greater pleasure, try the Venus Butterfly technique, or stimulating her clitoris and her G-spot at the same time. ✦

Things You Should Never Say to a Woman

1. Did you come yet?
2. Are you almost there?
3. Are you close?
4. How much longer do you need?
5. Does it always take you this long?

Even the best lover can become irritating if he doesn't pay attention to his partner. Here is my list of the ten most irritating things men do in bed:

1. Leaving your socks or shoes on. Forget what you learned from watching porn. If you are one of those guys who tends to rush getting undressed in the throes of passion, take your socks off first and stash them far, far away from her sensitive nose. Otherwise, try to undress as slowly as you can, and remember to remove your pants last.

2. Answering your cell phone. Cell phone use during intercourse seems to be at an all-time high. According to a BBDO Worldwide survey, 15 percent of Americans have interrupted sex to answer a cell phone call. To resist the urge to drop her breast for your ringing phone, turn it off before you begin foreplay. This is particularly true if your mother has a tendency to check up on you during the day. If she is likely to call, make sure to turn off your answering machine as well.

3. Engaging in small talk. Women love vocal, erudite men, but during intercourse is not the time to show off your gregariousness. So quit that chitchat and ditch the tautological demagoguery about the origin of the universe. The only thing you should be talking about is how much she turns you on and how great it feels to be inside her.

4. Watching anything other than her. This includes sports broadcasts. To avoid the temptation of staring at the TV, turn it off; better yet, remove it from your bedroom. A study by an Italian sexologist has found that couples who have a TV set in their bedroom have sex only half as often as those who don't. Other frequent transgressions include checking a clock or observing your pecs or beer belly in the mirror.

You are supposed to be looking at your woman (preferably in her eyes), and that means forgetting everything else. If you feel yourself getting distracted, try to redirect your attention by practicing mindfulness—staying in the moment by turning all of your senses to your current experience. Focus on the softness of her skin, the aroma of her hair, and the sounds of her moans.

5. Drooling on her (or spitting globs of saliva on her face). You can use your saliva as a moisturizer on her genitals, but keep it away from her face. It's gross, and she won't care if you've seen it in some adult movie.

6. Collapsing two seconds after your climax. In your defense, there is a physiological reason that men feel sleepy after orgasm. This is because the postclimactic blood rush depletes the muscles of energy-producing glycogen, leaving them feeling physically drained. Glycogen loss also triggers the release of adenosine, which acts as a messenger to the cells, triggering sleep. Because men have more muscle mass than women, men are more likely to feel sleepy just when their partners are yearning for some après-sex cuddling. But, just like you rose above your physiology's tendency to reach orgasm in two to five minutes, you can rise above this sleepiness reflex. Put some energetic dance music on the stereo or practice lovemaking in a place where you are unlikely to doze off, like on the kitchen counter. Whatever it takes, give your partner the romancing she needs while she is cooling down from the heat of your manly passion.

7. Mentioning the sexual skills of other women. Don't ever, ever talk about other women while making love. Women particularly resent you mentioning your ex-girlfriends or comparing your current experience to any you've had with another woman. Needless to say, consider any reference to a concurrent wife or girlfriend to be a total taboo. There might be an occasional exception, such as when she asks you to imagine having a threesome with Angelina Jolie or some other woman who turns her on. But otherwise, the rule is: when her panties come off, she is the only woman in the world for you.

8. Turning sex into stand-up comedy. You might be a potential winner at amateur night at your local Comedy Store, but forget about giggling, snickering, laughing, or telling jokes while making love. While women love a good sense of humor, and it's a great seduction tool, being silly or laughing can hamper her arousal and trivialize the sexual experience for her, so lose your humor with your clothes. You can pick it up again during postcoital bliss—after you've told her how great it was for you.

9. Using infantile pet names for body parts. Call a clit a clit, and a vagina a vagina, not a wee-wee. She doesn't care what you call your penis when you're masturbating or telling guy jokes with your buddies, or what your mother called it when she was changing your diapers. She wants to feel that she is a grown-up woman experiencing mature lovemaking with a real Prince Charming, and not a little girl "playing doctor." Sex is an adult activity, so grow up before engaging in it.

10. Forgetting about your physiological differences. She is not a RealDoll made to withstand 250 pounds of pressure, nor is her vagina ready to receive pillow-pounding thrusts from the first moment of contact. A woman's vagina is designed to receive maximum stimulation in its outer one to two inches and to expand (through a process called "tenting") to receive deeper and harder thrusts as her arousal progresses. So starting slowly, shallowly, and gently allows her to enjoy it much more—and prevents you from climaxing too soon—and also gives her time to work up to those heavy hip slammers.

Alternating positions, putting her on top for a time or going sideways or doggie style, keeps her from feeling crushed or unable to contribute to your lovemaking. Remembering that a woman takes longer to arouse and reach orgasm—and learning to be patient and gentle, and to hold back until she is ready—is not only good manners, it is what makes a man a lover.

So now you're fully stocked with all the information you'll need to know to keep your reputation as the best lover she's ever had.

Twenty

Size and Hardness: Getting Over Penis Issues

HOW TO GET OVER THE SIZE ISSUE

Women say it's not how much men have, but what we do with it. How many things can we do with it? What is it, Cuisinart? It's got two speeds: forward and reverse. —RICHARD LENI

You got your Frappuccino honey in your bedroom, and you worked her up into a sexual frenzy by delaying intercourse, stimulating all of her moan zones, and giving her incredible oral sex. You are about to take your drawers off, when the panic sets in: "What will she think of HIM?" You feel your shriveled member shiver in response to the possibility of being judged. This is the moment of truth, you think.

And you are not alone. Men are universally concerned with the size of their penis, wondering whether it measures up to those of other males, and whether it is capable of satisfying a woman. So does size really matter? The answer is a qualified no. Penile size is to men what breast size is to women—a part of the anatomy that has an effect on self-esteem that is actually disproportionate to its importance, at least as far as sexual satisfaction is concerned. As you will see, chances are your penis is average in size, and an average penis is perfectly fine for the majority of hot women.

Even though the length, width, and shape of the penis varies substantially, ranging from as small as only a few centimeters long to the longest one on record, which measured in at 14 inches, 88 percent of all men have penises between 5 to 7 inches long when erect. This is an adequate size for 90 percent of all women. Indeed, the average woman's vagina is only about 3 inches long, or about 4.5 inches long when fully aroused, and 2.4 inches in diameter. To accomodate a longer or thicker penis, it can stretch to fit; however, such stretching does not necessarily increase a woman's pleasure. Moreover, a long penis is often uncomfortable, as it tends to hit the cervical area, which most women don't find pleasurable. A longer penis also tends to be more floppy (less rigid) than a shorter one due to the greater blood volume needed to fill it out.

Penis girth has a higher correlation with female sexual satisfaction than penis length. Because the majority of vaginal nerve endings are located at the entrance of the vagina, wide penises with a pronounced, mushroom-like corona may be more adept at stimulating these nerves. However, wide penises are definitely not comfortable for oral and anal interactions. And again, the majority of penises are between 3 and 6 inches in girth, while an average vaginal circumference is about 2.4 inches. Whereas most vaginas can stretch to fit a thicker penis, many women find such stretching uncomfortable, particularly if they are not fully aroused.

Does it mean that penis size does not matter at all? No. It would be fallacious to assert that penis size has absolutely no effect on female satisfaction. A smaller penis (below 3 inches when erect) might fail to sufficiently stimulate some women, while an extremely long penis (above 7 inches) might make deep penetration painful. In addition, some women may prefer larger penises for reasons other than sexual satisfaction. Just like some men find very large breasts to be a turn-on, some women find large penises to be visually arousing, regardless of the practical implications of size. But remember, while most guys will stare at a woman with huge bazookas, they will actually prefer dating a woman with an average-size chest—and the same goes for women and penises. She might be wowed by a huge penis yet actually prefer a lover with an average-size one.

Of all the centerfolds I have interviewed, only one has emphasized the importance of the guy's penis for her arousal. She also admitted that she is only able to climax from intercourse. A majority of the centerfolds rated oral skills as more important to their sexual satisfaction than penis size (6.5 out of 10 was the mean importance of the penis size, and 8 out of 10 was the mean importance of oral skills). Pet of the Year Julie Strain said, "Penis size is not important to me because it is not how I come." So a long, agile tongue (a la Gene Simmons) probably gets higher rating scores from hot women than a long penis does!

Of course, in addition to being a sexual object, your penis is a symbol of virility, dominance, and masculine power. From that perspective, you might worry not so much about its ability to satisfy your hottie but about how it looks compared to those of other males she has been with. Perhaps you first became anxious about the size of your penis when you compared your undeveloped phallus to that of your father or older brother. Or maybe you used to look down at your own penis while comparing it to those of other boys in the locker room. Your anxiety might have become intensified by the visual effect called *foreshortening*. Every man sees his own penis in a *foreshortened view because looking down on it makes the penis appear shorter than it is.* That is why when he compares his penis to those of other men in a shower or changing room, his penis does not fare well in comparison. To get a better estimate of your penile size, look at yourself in the mirror instead of looking down.

Moreover, although women may talk about being thrilled by seeing the penis of a well-hung stud, in reality, the size of the relaxed or flaccid penis does not really matter, because during an erection, the penis may increase to several times its flaccid size. About 90 percent of all men have penises that range from 3 to 5 inches when flaccid. But some guys with below-average flaccid penises end up with above-average erections. These guys, or "growers," prove that an erection is the great equalizer.

Has she had bigger ones? No matter how curious you are, never, ever ask a hot woman how your penis compares to those of other lovers she has had. You will come across as an insecure chump, and she will never tell you the truth anyway. Instead, no matter what you are packing, carry it with pride. How can you expect her to like your penis if you don't fully accept it yourself? If you are overweight and have a belly, losing weight will make you appear more endowed (some claim that for every 35 pounds you gain, your stomach engulfs an extra inch of your penis). Shaving the genital area will also make your penis stand out and look larger. If you are tired of shaving, many hair removal centers service men who want permanent genital hair removal. Finally, taking your time during foreplay to cultivate your maximum erection will also make it appear larger when you finally reveal it to her.

Remember, even a below-average-sized penis can perform more than adequately when attached to a sensitive and skillful lover. Only 30 percent of women consistently achieve orgasms through intercourse, and the majority of women require additional clitoral stimulation to achieve orgasms. Learning how to achieve positions that maximize contact with her clitoris or that achieve maximum G-spot stimulation will put you far above most lovers she has ever had.

Even if your penis is on the small side, it may be superior in other ways to other penises she has had. It might taste better because you follow my nutrition advice (below). It might have smoother, softer skin than most or have a pronounced corona, or it might curve in a way that delivers her greater pleasure. Penises that curve upward are perfectly suited for stimulating the G-spot (except for an extreme curvature, which cannot affect penetration of a vagina and which is possibly a sign of Peyronie's disease). I once had a lover who was extremely self-conscious about his penis, which he considered crooked, as it had a pronounced downward bent. But once I showed him how to utilize his curvature to please a woman, he was no longer unhappy with his penis! In the doggy-style position he was able to give me absolutely the most powerful G-spot orgasms. What he considered to be a defect turned out to be a rare, delicious advantage!

What is far more important than the size is "the fit" between the couple, as anatomical compatibility can make a difference. Petite women often dislike the feel of a large penis, and some bigger women or those used to more filling stimulation sometimes prefer the larger ones. In my own experience, there is definitely a big difference in how well you match with some partners; some guys I felt literally merged with, and with others it seemed to require some effort to find a comfortable position for penetration. So if you really want to get her feedback, ask her what she thinks of how you fit together.

Finally, because every penis is attached to a man, when a woman feels passionate and turned on by a man, she is likely to imbue him with positive characteristics and perceive his penis as larger than it really is. Although love may not always be blind, infatuation always is. One of the guys I had the biggest crush on had a smaller-than-average penis. Besides, if you have followed my advice in the previous chapters, by now she is falling head over heels for you.

TIP #27: Tell yourself that penis size doesn't matter all that much—chances are, you are average, and average size is more than enough for an average woman. Any time you compare yourself, look at yourself in the mirror, not down, to avoid the foreshortening effect. To get your penis to look bigger, lose weight, shave your genital area, and cultivate maximum erection. Remind yourself that while size doesn't matter, fit does, and that you will be more compatible with some hotties than with others. You should never ask a woman questions about your size, such as, Is it big enough for you? Can you feel me inside? Have you had bigger ones? or Do you wish I was bigger? ✦

Myth Rebuffed: HOT WOMEN ONLY WANT TO SLEEP WITH WELL-ENDOWED MEN.

In fact, nothing could be further from the truth. Although women do comment on the guy's size, especially if he doesn't have much else to offer besides being well-endowed, none of the women I have interviewed picked their men on the basis of that quality alone. As a matter of fact, most of the centerfold's boyfriends are average, rather than well-endowed.

How to Overcome Performance Anxiety

I am going to Iowa for an award. Then I'm appearing at Carnegie Hall, it's sold out. Then I'm sailing to France to be honored by the French government. I'd give it all up for one erection.
—Groucho Marx

You have gotten over your worry about your penis size, and you are about to penetrate your Frappuccino hottie. She is wet, ready, and willing—no, beyond willing—she is begging you to plunge your penis into her. There is only one problem—HE decides not to cooperate. "Please, don't do this to me, not now!" you silently beg HIM. But the more you beg him, the more unenthusiastically he responds. What's a guy to do?!

For once, you need to stop this silent power struggle with your penis. Your erection is not under your willful muscular or cognitive control, and you absolutely cannot will an erection. As a matter of fact, trying to do so often backfires, as it escalates anxiety and anger, and other emotions incompatible with erectile response. What you need to do immediately is to stop trying. As Barbara Keesling[63] put it, "A watched pot never boils . . . and a watched penis never hardens."

Now listen to your inner self-talk. Are you working yourself into a panic by telling yourself, *This is awful! I must get it up or she will think I am a total loser! What if something is wrong with HIM, and I'll never ever get an erection again?! I am impotent!!!* Identify your negative cognitions and cognitive distortions, such as awfulizing, musturbation, exaggerating, mind-reading, labeling, and generalizing. Then actively rebut these thoughts by telling yourself, *This is not a big deal, it's just a temporary equipment malfunction!*

Check yourself for signs of anxiety, which include rapid and shallow breathing, a jumpy stomach and/or muscle tension in your thighs and abdomen. Take deep breaths and try to relax your leg muscles. Tightening the leg muscles is often responsible for erectile problems. This phenomenon is called "the pelvic steal syndrome," whereby tightening the leg muscles steals blood away from the penis. Make sure you are not tightening your muscles when you feel that you are going softer. Tightening your pelvic or anal sphincter muscles might make you feel as if you are pumping up your erection, but it actually causes your erection to go down. Instead, try to relax your muscles, even if it feels counterintuitive, and your erection will most likely return. To consciously remind yourself to relax your legs, give yourself a very light tap or pinch on the legs every time you feel them tighten.

The next step is to stop focusing on the sensations in your penis. This is called spectatoring, or vigilant preoccupation, a term coined by Masters and Johnson, which means you are thinking when you should be feeling or experiencing. Observing your penis, wondering how hard it is going to get, and ruminating over your sexual response are all examples of spectatoring. If you catch yourself thinking, *Am I going to get as hard as I do during masturbation? I bet it won't get very hard. Uh-oh, I think I feel it going down!* you need to shut down your overactive mind. Tell yourself that it is totally normal not to be as hard as you sometimes get because it is your first time with this hottie, and most women are very understanding of that. Remind yourself that sex is not a performance—it is an enjoyable activity—and if your penis does not feel like performing right now, it is OK.

Your next step is to focus on touching your partner. Feel the texture and temperature of her skin, pay complete attention to the point of contact between your skin and hers. You can also attune yourself to her smells and sounds. Think of all the things that you find arousing about her, and if that doesn't help, avail yourself of your nastiest sexual fantasy. That should get HIS attention, but if it doesn't don't fret. Tell your hottie you are not feeling your best today and offer to cuddle for a while—an offer she will likely accept. And remember, if you have been delaying intercourse all along, you can always say that you are not quite ready yet.

Your other option is to attempt penetration with a semi-rigid erection. Many men believe that they have to have a rock-hard penis in order to penetrate a woman, but that is a fallacy. According to Dr. Zilbergeld, the author of *The New Male Sexuality*, the popularization of porn films led many men and women to internalize the "fantasy model of sex," which portrays erections as automatic, hard as steel, and under willful control of their owners. In reality, an erection is anything but—a penis has a mind of its own, and the man can never will his penis to become hard;

the harder he tries, the softer his penis becomes. However, an erection does not have to be rock-hard to achieve penetration. Often, a softer penis can be made hard enough for penetration by gripping it firmly near its base, squeezing, and pulling it back to force the blood into the shaft. Once the penis is inserted in the vagina, it often becomes sufficiently hard to accomplish intercourse. As a matter of fact, that is what many male porn stars do, as Ron Jeremy once demonstrated to me. (Yes, he actually pulled out his penis and showed me how he can make a soft penis semi-hard by gripping it firmly and pushing blood into it. And no, I did not sleep with him!)

Chances are HE will eventually cooperate and you will have no problems giving your hottie the pounding of her life. However, if you continue to experience erection problems, even in situations that are not stressful or novel, you might be developing an erectile dysfunction, or ED. It is estimated that ED affects about 10 percent of American males (10 to 15 million men). About 85 percent of male impotence is due to physical causes, about 10 to 15 percent results from psychological causes. Physical impotence can result from injury, heart disease, prostate cancer, diabetes, liver failure, alcoholism, side effects from smoking or drugs, to name just a few. In most cases, physical causes of impotence are caused by endothelial dysfunction, which reduces or prevents blood flow or nerve impulses to the penis, but impotence can also be a result of lifestyle choices. Don't be frightened—it does not mean that you will have to turn to Viagra to get a hard-on from now on! Sometimes small lifestyle modifications, such as working out, flossing (yes, it's true!), reducing smoking and alcohol consumption, and improving your diet can greatly improve your erectile capacity. Men with more pervasive and persistent impotence should seek help from a doctor or sex therapist. There are numerous treatments for ED. The American Medical Association estimates that 95 percent of ED cases can be successfully treated with one of the many available options.

TIP #28: If you tend to go soft due to performance anxiety, make sure to relax. Tightening leg muscles sometimes steals blood away from the penis, a phenomenon called the "pelvic steal syndrome." Take deep, diaphragmatic breaths and stop spectatoring, or watching your erection. Reframe your negative cognitions by telling yourself that "what goes down will come up." Meanwhile, ease your performance pressure by focusing on her pleasure. If your erectile problems continue beyond novel situations, get a medical checkup. ✦

How to Last as Long as You Want

She was a lovely girl. Our courtship was fast and furious: I was fast and she was furious.   —Max Kaufman

I once made love for an hour and fifteen minutes, but it was the night the clocks are set ahead.   —Garry Shandling

You are pumping away, and your Frappuccino hottie is obviously enjoying herself. As your excitement is rising and rising, you find yourself getting closer and closer to the golden gates of ecstasy. Just at the point of no return, she cries out, "Don't come yet!" But it is too late . . . you have already shot your load.

One of the most frequent complaints that women have is that their partners come too fast. In fact, the average time the American male lasts during intercourse before climaxing is about 4 minutes. Women, on the other hand, take between 15 to 30 minutes to reach a climax. Obviously, both men and women would be happier if men could last longer in bed.

Nothing impresses a hottie more than a guy who can last until she tells him that it is OK to climax. I remember when several Pets and I were watching the taping of an adult film. The male porn stars were able to stop and start their pumping action on cue from the director and ejaculated only after the director told them to do so. Needless to say, we were absolutely blown away by that degree of ejaculatory control. Yet learning to delay ejaculation is one of the hardest things to do for many men.

Most men try to diminish their arousal by distracting themselves with nonsexual thoughts, such as baseball scores or job-related issues. Whereas this works for some men, most find that their arousal still "sneaks up" on them, and as much as an excited utterance from their woman puts them back into arousal and over the top. Others try to think of truly negative experiences, such as death or taxes, but that just makes lovemaking a less enjoyable experience. For some men pinching themselves or biting the pillows helps to bring their level of arousal down and delay orgasm.

One of the first things you should do if you want to learn to last longer is to change your autoerotic style—and I am not talking about your adoration for your automobile here! Most guys do not realize that the way they masturbate has a direct effect on their performance with women. In fact, most sex therapists believe that premature ejaculation is caused by the man's early, furtive sexual experiences—rushed so as to avoid detection. This hectic rush conditions guys to climax as quickly as possible. Similarly, if you are used to fast masturbation, it will often translate into problems during intercourse. You have essentially conditioned yourself to rapid orgasm, and now you have to work against a learned response. In fact, sex therapists list "abusive masturbation" as one of the main reasons for erection and ejaculation problems during intercourse.

So stop thinking, *I've got five minutes before my boss calls me in, enough time for a quick jack-off!* Think of your self-love sessions as a training ground for intercourse; if you can learn to pace yourself during masturbation, you will have an easy time translating that pace into intercourse. Set the time when you are not going to be rushed, and the place where you will not be disturbed, and masturbate with dry hands almost to the point of ejaculation, then stop. Do it three times, then permit yourself to ejaculate. Once you achieve this measure of control, do it with a wet hand, which tends to feel closer to a vaginal environment. If you train yourself to require longer time and harder stimulation to climax during masturbation, that association is likely to translate itself into intercourse.

In fact, this is how most male porn stars learn to be so proficient at controlling their ejaculation. As one of the male porn stars I interviewed responded, "I just sit there on my days off, playing with myself—I get myself close to coming, then back off and let myself go soft, then work myself up again, then back down again. I don't let myself ejaculate for hours until I get hungry, then I just count til three and let myself come." This guy was obviously not a rocket scientist, but he knew that his livelihood depended on his ability to withhold his orgasm, so he learned to identify his states of arousal.

This technique of identifying one's states of arousal is called "peaking" in sex therapy. Practicing "peaking" exercises is the primary way of achieving ejaculatory control. Peaking is learning to recognize your arousal states by slowly elevating your level of arousal, then reducing stimulation when orgasm approaches. Once you learn to recognize that approaching point of no return, or ejaculatory inevitability, you will know when to slow down and decrease the sensations you are feeling from intercourse, thereby reducing your arousal, and delaying ejaculation. For some guys, lengthening and slowing down their thrusts is enough to bring their arousal down, while others need to stop or withdraw to keep them from orgasming. You can slow down and focus on kissing and caressing her, or you can withdraw and go down on her for a while before resuming your thrusting. Either way, I am sure she will love the attention!

Another proven way of gaining ejaculatory control is by strengthening your pelvic muscles.

You might have heard of Kegeling, or pelvic exercises for women. Men, too, benefit from PC muscle exercises in many ways, particularly in the area of ejaculatory control. To locate your PC muscle, lightly place two fingers behind your testicles. Now imagine that you are urinating and want to stop the flow by squeezing the internal muscle. Practice squeezing and relaxing this muscle group at least twenty-five times in three sessions per day. Once you develop control over this muscle, you can squeeze your PC muscles several times until you feel your arousal go down.

What made me a believer in the power of PC muscles was watching the *Puppetry of the Penis* production, where two bare-ass-naked performers show off the ancient art of Australian Genital Origami. These guys use their PC muscles to twist and contort their penises into unusual shapes and even to retrieve their penises into the pelvic cavity. If that can be done, using PCs to delay ejaculation should be a breeze! The trick is to be able to identify the beginning of the orgasm phase when the seminal fluid (or "pre-cum," in lay terms) appears and muscular rigidity begins to set in right before the release of tension. *At the point of impending orgasm and before the point of no return, you must contract the pelvic muscle with sufficient pressure to be able to stop the ejaculation.* A small amount of sperm might still seep out, but you should still be very aroused and able to continue penile stimulation. The best way to learn this by masturbatory practices, when you can pace yourself and learn to identify the stages of your sexual response cycle.

Another way to maintain an erection after an orgasm is the Taoist way—by pressing an acupuncture point located halfway between the anus and the scrotum. This point is known as the Jen-Mo acupuncture point, and when pressed with a finger, this point feels as if there is a small indention or hole in that location. According to the Tao, when the Jen-Mo point is pressed just prior to an anticipated ejaculation, the ejaculation can be reversed into an improved orgasm and the seamen is recycled from the full prostate and reabsorbed into the blood in the process called "injaculation." Done this way, the man still feels the pleasurable sensations that come with the pumping of the prostate, and he still experiences an orgasm, but he continues to experience an erection. If you want to try this, at the moment just before you are ready to ejaculate, simply reach around behind your buttocks and locate the point. Press it hard enough so that the semen is not allowed travel out of the prostate and through the urethra. Taoists also recommend prostate massage for men who want to learn to last longer. If you are interested in Taoist techniques, there are numerous books written on the subject.

Another way to maximize your ability to last is to choose sexual positions that put the least pressure on you, allowing you to focus on her pleasure. Side-by-side and woman-on-top positions allow you to slow down stimulation when it becomes too intense. Another position that should maximize your ability to last and her ability to orgasm is *coital alignment technique,* or CAT.[64]

This is sometimes described as "riding higher in the saddle," as it involves the man sliding his pelvis higher on the woman's body so that his pubic bone (the horizontal bone immediately above the penis) directly contacts her clitoris. To achieve this effect, you must not only move your pelvis three to four inches higher on her body but you should also shorten your stroke, rocking forward and backward rather than fully withdrawing and thrusting. Each forward and backward movement should be only far enough to rub her clitoris with your pubic bone.

The obvious significance of this position is that it provides maximum clitoral stimulation for the woman and helps her achieve orgasm. In addition, it changes the angle of the penis in a way to maximize friction on top of the penis and at the tip. Full insertion is likely to be difficult or impossible, due to the angle of the penis. Prolonged use of this position might not provide you with enough stimulation to keep your erection; therefore, it might be necessary to switch to standard missionary from time to time to maintain it.

Whereas these techniques work for most men, there is a small percentage of men who appear to be unable to delay their ejaculatory response, no matter how much training or practice they get. There is some research indicating a genetic predisposition to premature ejaculation in those men. For them, SSRI inhibitors, such as Prozac and Zoloft, have been effective in delaying ejaculation.

If you are one of the men who cannot seem to last longer than 5 minutes, do not despair. As I have mentioned above, most women achieve orgasms through oral sex, not intercourse. And while some women love a long session of penile thrusting (I am partial to men who can last more than 10 minutes because I relish the feeling of being merged together), others get sore easily and prefer shorter intercourse. While Pet of the Year Julie Strain loves being pleasured orally, she is not fond of prolonged intercourse: "Come quick or better not call me again! The best time is five minutes, I don't want to be stretched out and sore. I want to go back to watching TV together!"

TIP #29: If you tend to fire off quickly, the first thing you should do is change your masturbatory style from quick to slow and deliberate; practicing peaking and going soft, a form of stop-start exercises. Once you learn to distinguish your point of no return, try to slow down and decrease stimulation by focusing on pleasing her, or changing sexual positions. Woman-on-top and side-by-side positions should allow you to last longer. Exercising your PC muscles will also permit you to gain greater control over your ejaculatory reflex. You can also try squeezing the shaft of your penis or pressing on the indentation in your perineum area when you are getting close to ejaculating. Finally, if none of the techniques described here are working, you can get prescription meds that would permit you to last longer. ✦

I've listed a few more ways to last longer in bed, starting from the least effective quick fixes to long-term solutions.

1. Masturbate beforehand. Most men orgasm sooner when they haven't climaxed in a long time. So give yourself some self-love while checking out our sexy Pets before bedding your honey. Practice slow self-love, working yourself up, then allowing yourself to go soft before resuming again. Just make sure to conceal the evidence of your auto-eroticism—lest you have to use it as hair gel, like the protagonist of *There's Something About Mary*.

2. Numb your penis, or put on a cock ring or a condom. These are "quick fixes" that don't work for many guys. Using a desensitizing cream might keep you from getting overexcited, but it will give you a numb penis and might reduce her sensation as well. Similarly, many guys report that decreasing the amount of sensation by wearing a condom or trapping the blood in it with a penis ring helps them last longer. If you want to make her really happy, don a "One Shot" Vibrating penis ring, which has a tiny vibrating egg designed to stimulate her clitoris.

3. Visualize your ugly neighbor. Those of you who have a fertile imagination can use the power of visualization to stave off the upcoming orgasm. For some guys, thinking of something that is the opposite of "sexy," such as a fat, bitchy boss, or something sad, such as the death of a loved one, works in bringing down their arousal level. Others replay hockey games or chess moves in their minds. Some guys swear by these techniques, whereas others complain that they end up going totally limp.

4. Have an alcoholic drink. Alcohol slows down all of your reflexes, along with your ejaculatory reflex. But don't use this technique too often, or you will develop a tolerance for alcohol and will need greater and greater amounts of it. Keep doing that and you may pass out on top of her without ever ejaculating.

5. Check your prostate. Research shows that up to 50 percent of severe premature ejaculation is aggravated by an inflamed prostate. So don't allow your fear of anal exams to prevent you from seeing your doctor and checking out your prostate health.

6. Try Deferol. Deferol Climax Control Supplement is an all-natural, clinically proven supplement that allows men greater climax control by regulating serotonin and dopamine levels, which are both implicated in lack of ejaculatory control (www.deferol.com).

7. Use the "squeeze technique." This technique was developed by Masters and Johnson to be used on a man by his female partner, but some men report using it on themselves successfully. When you sense you are about to experience an orgasm, squeeze the shaft of your penis between your thumb and two fingers. Apply light pressure just below the head of your penis for about 20 seconds, then let go and resume sexual stimulation. I've seen porn stars use this technique to last longer.

8. Use the "stop and start technique." This technique basically involves slowing down or holding off just before ejaculation. This allows the level of arousal to subside, giving more preclimax control.

9. Move to the music. Choose a piece of instrumental music with a very slow beat and pay attention to the beat of the music. Then start to stroke slowly, switching your focus back and forth from the feelings in your penis to the music. See if you can keep up with the music by matching one stroke per beat or one stroke per two beats.

10. Get prescription medication. For some men, Viagra and other similar drugs help prolong intercourse, because the men who take them continue to experience erections even after ejaculation. The use of SSRI inhibitors commonly used to treat depression and anxiety, such as Prozac and Zoloft, effectively delay ejaculation. However, do not take these every day—only on days when you are planning to have sex.

Twenty-one

EMO and CAT:
Getting Her Off in Multiple Ways

Now I know what I have been faking all these years.
——GOLDIE HAWN in *Private Benjamin*

When a female friend of mine casually mentioned to me several years ago that her new lover brought her numerous orgasms by stimulating her manually, I scoffed. I knew that Masters and Johnson discovered that some women are capable of having more than one orgasm during a sexual session, but I also knew that few of my female friends were multiorgasmic. Yet, the research showed that while male ejaculation is almost always followed by a sharp drop in arousal, a woman's arousal continues to remain moderately high after she has climaxed. Masters and Johnson called this state of continuing arousal "the plateau"; in their research, they found some women could enjoy up to twenty successive vaginal orgasms from continuous stimulation. Indeed, later research by the same team discovered a state called *status orgasmus,* or "sustained orgasm." In particular, one female subject they examined was able to sustain an orgasm for forty-three seconds with twenty-five separate contractions.

However, not every woman has the ability to achieve such an orgasmic nirvana, either because of physiological or psychological factors. The multiorgasmic ability is very uncommon among young women; it is mostly a learned response. This corresponds to the research showing that a woman's sexual desire actually peaks in her early thirties and that having a vaginal delivery often increases sexual responsiveness. Nevertheless, with patience and practice, many women can learn to have more than one orgasm during a lovemaking session, particularly with a patient lover dedicated to her pleasure.

Training the object of your desires to experience multiple orgasms or a lengthy sustained one will ensure that she will want you in her bed again and again. Since it is likely that she has never experienced such a thrill before encountering you, it will mark you as a nonpareil lover; moreover, it will convince her that you are truly attentive to her pleasure and to her as a person. Succeed at this, and you should be able to write your own ticket for future sexual opportunities with your chick; and if you are looking for something more than just sex, it will help you realize that dream as well. So how do you go about it?

As noted above, there are really two types of multiple orgasms. One is the *sequential multiple,* where separate orgasms are experienced two to ten minutes apart, with the woman's arousal level declining only to the plateau level and then resuming its climb to a repeat orgasm. The other type is the *serial orgasm,* where a woman experiences orgasms one after another without any drop in arousal between them. The sequential multiples are often the product of first attaining clitoral orgasm from oral or digital sex and then moving to vaginal intercourse, where further orgasms occur. In some situations, following up a clitoral orgasm achieved through lighter pressure by hand or mouth stimulation with harder stimulation from a sex toy can produce a second clitoral orgasm. On the other hand, serial multiples are almost always vaginal orgasms.

The key to producing sequential multiple orgasms appears to be prolonged and varied stimulation. According to the Bodanskys, a couple who authored the book on the Extended Massive Orgasm (or EMO), the easiest way for a woman to experience a massive orgasm is through manual stimulation. They recommend that a woman position herself comfortably on her back with her legs bent and raised. Her partner should start by gently stroking her vulva, then slowly rubbing the knob of her clitoris with a lubricated finger, then adding his middle finger, varying speed and pressure depending on what feels good. He can use his thumb at the same time to put some pressure on her vaginal opening. When the woman feels that the orgasm is approaching, she should let her partner know so that he can slow down. He should then use short, quick strokes to bring her back up. After this, he should add more lubrication, make a V shape with the pointer and middle fingers of his other hand, and insert into the vaginal opening. He should apply pressure with an in-and-out motion at eleven and one o'clock, experimenting with different speeds and pressures. After a while, he should change the position of his fingers vaginally, stimulating at three and nine o'clock, and pushing downward with two fingers at six o'clock. This technique can lead to an extended orgasm in some women, such as Vera Bodansky, who demonstrates her own one-hour orgasms during her workshops.

Finally, to give her a serial vaginal orgasm through intercourse, you need to be able to prolong intercourse, varying your stimulation both in penile angle and in speed and depth of thrust. This means first learning the techniques discussed above for withholding your climax. Once you can confidently last for as long as she wants you to, you can try to maximize the number of orgasms she enjoys while you are thrusting inside her. The easiest way to reach for multiples is to let her be on top first, where she can move in ways that maximize her pleasure. You can use your hands to massage her breasts and clitoris while she is riding you, or you can use a vibrator on her clitoris.

If she likes to have her man on top (which is my favorite position), you can modify the missionary position to increase her chances of climaxing in that position. The coital alignment technique, or CAT, which was described previously, is the best way to stimulate her clitoris though.

A variation on the CAT is "the female CAT," where the woman slides up slightly on the man's body until she can feel her clitoris rub against her lover's pubic bone; then she rocks in this position to maximize her clitoral stimulation. This position is even easier to attain than standard missionary CAT, as the woman can feel when her clitoris is in the right place and get there almost instantly, while the man might fumble around trying to get it right from the male-on-top position. For women who require clitoral stimulation in order to reach orgasm during intercourse, the CAT is the best way to do so.

The CAT could be alternated with another modification—"the raised hip missionary" position, where a pillow or a Liberator cushion is place under her buttocks to elevate her pelvis, thereby allowing for the optimal stimulation of her G-spot. Adding manual or vibrator stimulation, both clitorally and anally, has also been reported to enhance and prolong orgasms. Most of the hotties I interviewed love sex toys and enjoy when guys use them during sexual encounters. You can start by getting the new Trojan condom with a vibrating ring and observe her response. Should you ask her first before pulling out a sex toy or just do it? A majority of the centerfolds responded that you should ask before using the toy for the first time. Pet of the Year Jamie Lynn responded, "If I don't know him well, he should ask, but if it's not our first time, go for it." Pet Krista Ayne is enthusiastic about a guy buying her sex toys: "I think it's fun to use them—it adds something to sex. I would like it if a guy bought sex toys for me because I would know he is into trying new things and that it was important for him to please me." Julie Strain also loves sex toys, but she warns the guy not to use them without asking her first: "If I use them myself, jump right in! But don't bust out the bag out of your closet that you used on other people!" Pet Courtney Taylor also loves sex toys, but she stresses that "they must be an addition to the repertoire. As long as he is not using them so that he doesn't have to do as much work." So make sure to show her what you can do with your tongue and hands first before resorting to sex toys.

Try experimenting with various lubricants—scented, flavored, etc. Try getting her Zestra, a natural botanical oil that enhances arousal and orgasm in women—and men, too!

Achieving such multiple O's, whether by using the Bodanskys' approach, by working up to serial vaginal orgasms, or by adding sex toys is not something you can realistically expect to achieve the first night you spend with your honey. But since she is that hottie you have always dreamed of having, you will want her to return for many more such sessions—assuming you don't tire from her narcissism or her addictions to beauty treatments and clothes shopping. So it will usually further your plans to show her some books like the Bodanskys' or some online articles on the subject of multiple orgasms and have her thinking about it between dates. It will give her another reason not only to accept your invitations but also to hop into your bed whenever you ask. You can even use this during your presex dating stage, when you are withholding inter-course from her in order to cement her interest in you:

SHE: "Why won't you have sex with me, especially after we have been making out now for hours?"

YOU: "It's just that I think of sexual intercourse as a very pow-erful, intimate experience, and I always strive during sex to produce multiple, even extended serial orgasms for my part-ner. So she has to be a very special woman to share that goal and be willing to practice towards achieving it with me."

You can then give her some books or articles you have printed out from the Internet and let her think about them, and discuss them with you on subsequent dates. It's all a part of teasing and tantaliz-ing her mind, and raising her desire for you.

However, always remember that not all women are capable of achieving multiple O's, so always be ready to reassure her that if you don't succeed, there is nothing "wrong" with her. Both of you should treat the effort as fun, and no matter what success you have, she will always appreciate your trying, as it evidences your care for her pleasure and happiness. And like the medieval quests for the Holy Grail, there is much to enjoy in the striving for pleasure, too.

TIP #30: The way to get her to experience sequential multiple orgasms is by introducing prolonged and varied stimulation, whether by manipulating her vagina with your hands with the Bodansky method, combining manual and oral stimulation, or prolonging intercourse while choosing sexual positions that bring her the most consistent stimulation of her clitoris (with the CAT technique) or G-spot (with elevating her hips in the missionary position or doing her doggy style). ✦

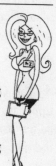

Her 8 Orgasmic Spots You Don't Want to Miss

As if finding the G-spot was not complicated enough, there appear to be other areas of the female genitals that have orgasmic capacity. Not all women respond to stimulation of these areas, but you should always try and see if your hottie is responsive. Begin with mons pubis and work your way down and in, observing her reactions on your way. If these zones are too confusing, stimulate her vagina in a clockwise fashion until you find her magical feel-good spots.

1. The mons pubis—a rounded fleshy protuberance situated over her pubic bones that becomes covered with hair during puberty. Some women prefer that you stimulate this area first before moving down to the clitoris.

2. The clitoris—a knoblike pleasure organ, which is located at the junction of the labia minora, above the opening of the urethra. Virtually every woman responds to clitoral stimulation, although some women prefer direct clitoral stimulation, while others prefer that you play with the clitoris through the clitoral sheath.

3. The U-spot—stands for the urethra, as it is located at the front entrance to the urethra, just underneath the clitoris, between the vaginal opening and the G-spot. To see if she likes her U-spot stimulated, put your thumb on the clitoral sheath and your forefinger inside the vagina and then rub them together in the "mo' money" gesture.

4. The G-spot—located 1.5 to 3 inches inside the vagina on the upper wall. When aroused it's about the size of a quarter and can be felt by inserting one or two fingers into the vagina and crooking them up in the "come here" gesture.

5. The E-zone—or epicenter, is located just above the cervix on the upper wall of the vagina, a few inches further than the G-spot. Some women experience "uterine" orgasms from stimulation of this area.

6. The AFE-zone—stands for the Anterior Fornix Erotic Zone. The fornix is the area surrounding the cervix, and the AFE-zone is located anterior to, or in front of, the fornix, about an inch or two up the rear side of the vaginal wall, opposite the G-spot.

7. The P-zone—the perineum is the area of skin between the vagina and the anus. Many women enjoy stimulation of this area, as it indirectly stimulates the anus.

8. The A-zone—or area all around the anus, is almost always a site of pleasure for a woman. Just because she likes her A-zone massaged does not mean she would be into anal sex, though.

Twenty-two

Fantasies:
Entering Her Secret Garden

Billy Crystal: That's it? A faceless guy rips off your clothes and that's the sex fantasy you've been having since you were twelve. Exactly the same?

Meg Ryan: Well, sometimes I vary it a little.

BC: Which part?

MR: What I am wearing.

—*When Harry Met Sally*

While giving her the greatest head she has ever received; lasting longer than any man she has been with; and helping her achieve multiple orgasms for the first time in her life should keep her coming back to your bed as often as you want, you don't want her—or you—to get bored by repeating the same things over and over. One good way to avoid that dismal result is to explore—and exploit—her sexual fantasies.

Exploring her fantasies has two distinct benefits. First, it keeps your sexual relationship fresh and new, helping you avoid any chance of boredom, and it helps keep it fun and varied, adding to your mutual bedroom enjoyment. But second, it also helps foster a higher degree of intimacy between you. As I have emphasized above, intimacy and connection are vitally important to a woman's sexual satisfaction, not to mention her ability to fall in love with a guy. Disclosing her deepest sexual fantasies to you, especially those which society might deem "wicked," means she feels you are worthy of a level of trust and intimacy that she might never have shared with another man. For this reason, you will want to exploit those disclosures, and the sexual play that follows them, to further the sense of "connectedness" that you want to build between you. This is certainly true if you are looking for a long-term relationship with the hottie you have induced to become your lover, but even if you are just looking for sex from her on a regular basis, developing your *sexual* intimacy will be the key to keeping her coming back for more.

What kind of fantasies are we talking about? For centuries it was widely believed that "normal" women did not have sexual fantasies. The seminal work that first publicized the private world of women was Nancy Friday's anthology of women's fantasies, *The Secret Garden,* and its several sequels. As illustrated in Friday's compendiums, and in a number of the studies that followed, a majority of men and women prefer similar fantasy themes. One of these pioneering studies of fantasy found that the following five fantasies are most common for both men and women: intercourse with a loved one, intercourse with a stranger, multiple partners of the opposite sex at the same time, doing things sexually that you would never do in reality, and being forced or forcing someone to have sex. "Intercourse with a loved partner" was found to be the most exciting fantasy for both men and women in a study conducted in the early '80s. Two other studies found that the two most popular fantasies for both men and women were being with another partner and reliving a previous sexual experience.

However, these studies also found that while men and women fantasize about similar sexual themes, the tone and style of their fantasies, and thus the way they dream them playing out, is dramatically different. Women's fantasies are more emotional, contextual, intimate, and romantic. Unlike men, women rely less on visual references and more on romantic outcomes and emotional feelings to fuel their sexual fantasies. For this reason, a woman's fantasies will likely have moments of affection and commitment within their content. Your fantasies probably run to imagining the specific sexual acts you would like to perform with your favorite centerfold, or how you would like to kiss or suck on her breasts. Most male fantasies are similar. However, your favorite centerfold's fantasies about you—assuming she has met you and you have snowed her with the techniques described in the preceding chapters—would be more likely to dwell on the emotions she felt when you touched her hand, or the way you couldn't take her eyes off her in her new, tight-fitting dress. If she does fantasize about having sex with you, her daydreams would likely focus on such things as how sweet your kisses felt to her and how dreamily content she felt in your arms after she climaxed.

Women are also more likely to feel conflicted about their sexual fantasies. According to research, about one in four people of both sexes feel strong guilt about their fantasies; however, the percentage of women with these guilt feelings is much higher. Most of us, but especially women, feel guilty fantasizing while making love to their partners because we consider such fantasies a form of symbolic betrayal or cognitive infidelity. Having sexual fantasies about someone other than our partner makes us question our integrity—how can we be in love with one person and thinking about another? The way most of us deal with this form of guilt is to repress it. In one study of college students, 22 percent of the female respondents and 8 percent of the male respondents said they usually try to repress the feelings associated with fantasy. People also feel guilty when their fantasy and personal ideology are in conflict. A strong and independent woman might feel guilty and ashamed about having fantasies of being dominated by an insensitive brute. People who have what they consider to be unusual or deviant fantasies might also feel guilt and shame about them—and might even fear that such fantasies would cause them to lose control or act out in socially unacceptable ways.

Moreover, research has shown that those who feel guilty over their sexual fantasies have sex less often and enjoy it considerably less. So if you want to explore your dream girl's sexual fantasies, you might need to help her get over any feelings of shame or guilt she might have about disclosing them. You can do that by convincing her that her fantasies are normal for many women and then encouraging her to accept them. Get some of Nancy Friday's books, *Penthouse Letters,* or other descriptive accounts of female fantasies, show her that other women share her desires and daydreams, and explain that reputable scientific research shows that these fantasies are quite normal. You can use these books to explore her fantasies also, by telling her you read about them and asking for her thoughts on them: "I read in *The Secret Garden* that many women fantasize about being tied up and stimulated to multiple orgasms. Do you ever have such fantasies?"

Other ways to discover her fantasies include renting and watching a mainstream film or DVD portraying those fantasies, such as *The Bitter Moon* by Roman Polansky, which shows a couple engaging in steamy acts of mild S&M, voyeurism, and exhibitionism, or *Wild Things,* which portrays a hot threesome with Denise Richards. Or you might rent a DVD of the TV show *Nip/Tuck,* which features just about every taboo fantasy—such as sex with a transvestite, partner pretending to be a prostitute, etc.—and watch it together. During the show, you can watch her reactions and get a feel for how she is responding to it, then discuss it together afterwards. You can also encourage her to disclose her fantasies by agreeing to "trade" her disclosure for one of yours, or by playing adult versions of "Truth or Dare" and other games requiring disclosure. If you need to overcome her reluctance to talk about a particular fantasy, you can go on the Internet to explore them on websites and chat groups together, as that is a good first step in making the fantasy less frightening. The next step might be to introduce couples-oriented X-rated films that further explore her particular fantasies.

Another way to explore fantasies she is willing to reveal is by having the two of you each write down your sexual wishes and put them into a "sexual wish" basket, taking turns drawing them every night—either to talk about them or, better yet, perform them!

You should never push her into fulfilling a fantasy; instead, gently encourage her to further explore it. Even if she does not feel any guilt, repressed or otherwise, about having the fantasy, she might not want reality entering into her fantasy world—which is likely the world in which she masturbates. Also, remember that fantasies often lose their erotic appeal after they are brought into real experience, so if her fantasy is a particularly cherished one, she might want to keep it unfulfilled. However, when she expresses interest in fulfilling her fantasy, you should plan a way to carry it out. Fantasy fulfillment should be well planned out and discussed in advance, so you can make it as close to her daydreams as possible.

ENACTING THE SUBMISSION FANTASY

Women, by nature, want to be dominated.

—JAYNE MANSFIELD

Any reader of Nancy Friday's compendium of female sexual fantasies will be struck by how often they involve the woman being tied up, spanked, or otherwise "forced" to have sex. Research has suggested that over 40 percent of all women have had such fantasies and that it might even be more common, as many women might refuse to admit to such fantasies even with promises of anonymity. But the common misconception that these fantasies connote a desire to be raped misses the important details. In these fantasies, the woman imagines that her dominator is a sexually desirable man, that he is motivated by true passion that is aroused by her sexual attractiveness, and that he uses just enough force and stimulation to overcome her resistance and to promote her sexual pleasure. That is not "rape" in any sense of the word but consensual sex with a desirable and loving mate—the domination and discipline are only the means which are fantasized to bring about the desired climax. Read any of those "bodice ripper" romance novels that women buy, the ones with pirate captains abducting and using the heroines, or knights dueling with each other for her favors and then "having their way" with the heroines. All of them have the fantasy elements described above.

Most centerfolds I have interviewed enjoy surrender fantasies. Pet of the Year Jamie Lynn admits she likes being dominated, and Pet of the Month Erica Ellyson excitedly agrees: "Tie me up and blindfold me, baby, you can handle the rest." Centerfold Brea Lynn has never been tied up but she is enthusiastic about trying BDSM. Pet of the Year Runner-ups Courtney Taylor and Krista Ayne both love the mystery of surrender, and Krista is not shy about expressing her love of submission: "I was the one that asked for it!" But make sure to discuss her limits before trying BDSM with her. Playmate of the Month Charlotte Kemp warns against a guy going too far: "I love playful domination, anything more and I will shut down."

Knowing these things, how do you go about exploring these hidden—perhaps deeply hidden—fantasies in a responsible manner? First, you have to talk about them. You need to know exactly how she has fantasized these scenes and what limits she might have set on them. Perhaps she might have envisioned being bound and "tortured" sexually for hours, or spanked or whipped to tears and pleading before "giving in." Or perhaps she only imagined putting up a token resistance before the scene turned to purely sexual activities. The difference is monumental; you need to explore all the parameters of her fantasies—and yours.

Second, you need to give her the assurance that the scene will never go beyond her limits, no matter how helpless she is. You do this by giving her a "safe word" that will enable her, once she speaks it, to terminate the session immediately, plus your solemn promise to honor her safe word instantly.

Now that you know why and what is involved in her submission fantasies, how do you go about staging them? Simulated "rape" scenes are fairly easy. The setting, the mood, and the amount of pretended "force" she wants you to use are the key factors. Beyond that, they are just like any role-playing sexual game. Always remember, though, that even though you are playing a rapist, in her fantasies, the rapist is always a great guy at heart who will ultimately fall in love with her. His use of "force" is only triggered by the intensity of his desire for her delightful body, such that he cannot hold back or take "no" for an answer.

Bondage fantasies are also quite straightforward. You simply tie her up—to a bed, chair, or any handy object, or her body by itself—and then proceed to tease and torment her sexually, with feathers, fur, fingers, and whatever else your fertile imagination can come up with. Be sure to use soft bonds that won't bite into her skin. Bathrobe cords, neckties, or silk scarves work well, or you can buy some soft restraints. When you "have her where you want her," you can play with her body, using all of the techniques for arousing a woman discussed above: oral sex, multiple orgasms, and the like. When you are finished with the scene, make sure you let her know how much you enjoyed her body and her gift of submission. You are, after all, her Prince Charming—a sensitive but caring brute.

TIP # 31: Women's fantasies are more emotional, contextual, intimate, and romantic. Unlike men, women rely less on visual references and more on romantic outcomes and emotional feelings to fuel their sexual fantasies. Try discussing the following fantasies with her: intercourse with a loved one, intercourse with a stranger, multiple partners of the opposite sex at the same time, doing things sexually that you would never do in reality, and being forced or forcing someone to have sex. Then pick the one that appeals to her the most and role-play it with her. Most hotties fantasize about being overpowered by a sensitive but caring brute. ✦

Playing with Her Sexual Fantasies

HIT	MISS
Pretending to be her boss	Pretending to be her cousin
Talking like her favorite actor	Talking like her ex-husband
Wearing a mask to bed after warning her	Wearing a mask without warning her
Bringing home a girl she wants	Bringing home a girl you want
Forcing her to endure oral pleasuring	Forcing her to pleasure you orally
Doing her in the car	Doing her in Times Square

Top 6 Role-Play Scenarios

Short on role-play ideas? Try these popular and easy-to-re-create scenarios:

1. Doctor-patient. Playing doctor is not only for kids. Pretend your hottie is gravely ill and needs a full body exam to see what's wrong with her.

2. Boss-secretary. You have just hired a new secretary who wears short tight skirts, frequently drops your documents, then bends over at the waist to pick them up.

3. Teacher-student. You are a strict teacher who believes in corporal punishment, and she is a naughty student who deserves a good spanking. Take it from there.

4. Repairman-housewife. You are a hardworking plumber and she is a bored housewife looking for some action. Check her plumbing system as you bend her over that overflowing toilet.

5. **Police officer–driver.** Pretend to pull your hottie over, then slap some handcuffs on her and make her work her way out of that ticket.

6. **Sultan-concubine.** She is a new concubine in your large harem, and she needs to work extra hard for you to keep you from selling her.

Twenty-three

Anal, Threesomes, and Swallowing: Take Her to the Wild Side

Now that you have her satisfied above and beyond her wildest dreams, you can try taking her even further—to the fantasyland most men can only dream of, where hot women play with sex toys, swallow, have anal sex, and eagerly engage in ménages-a-trois with you and other hotties. And if you have followed my advice so far, chances are your hottie is willing to follow you to the ends of the earth because she trusts in your ability to bestow you with unprecedented pleasure.

> *Women are really not that exacting. They only desire one thing in bed. Take off your socks. And by the way—they're never going to invite their best girlfriend over for a threesome, so you can stop asking.*
> —DENNIS MILLER

THE BIG GULP AND HOW TO GET ONE (WHEN SHE'S GOING DOWN ON YOU)

The Shangri-la of oral sex for men is a girlfriend that swallows. Unfortunately, the majority of women do not fit swallowing into their vision of paradise. Some complain of the taste of semen; others can't contain the spurting love juice without gagging. What, then, does a man do to get his woman to give him the gift of a great gulping, sucking swallow while he shoots his load down her throat?

Fortunately for you, guys, 95 percent of the women I interviewed said they do swallow under the right circumstances. And most of them do it of their own accord. Pet of the Year Runner-up Courtney Taylor said that she would swallow "if I trust the guy and think it will be long term. I would never do it if a guy asks me to. That would be somewhat sadistic, because why would a guy care if you swallowed or not? I would just do it on my own to show the guy I don't think it is gross—that I like his taste." The taste of your semen has a lot to do with the girl's willingness to swallow, according to my survey, so make sure to heed my diet advice below if you want her to love the way you taste.

First, you need to make her want to do it, despite all her reservations and past experiences. When cuddling after sex, or at any other such romantic moments, mention that you find oral sex to provide the ultimate in sexual intimacy. Ask her to describe her greatest oral sex fantasy in prolonged detail, and promise to make it happen. (Of course, you'd better be prepared to follow through on this, or you will likely blow it, rather than get blown!) When you have gotten her thinking in this vein, she will likely ask how she can reciprocate, to get you to experience this intimacy with her. That's when you drop the load on her, figuratively of course, that for you, such intimacy can only be experienced when she swallows.

Give her the Tantric line about your semen being the carrier of your life energy, which you pour into her as your most intimate gift; and that you feel rejected and shamed when a woman spits it out. Build up this picture of Oriental mystical nirvana and rejection-if-not-swallowed with lines from the Kama Sutra or the Chinese "pillow books," but emphasize the symbolic meaning of the act of swallowing: acceptance and ingestion of the other's deepest, most intimate essence. Tears are a good thing to let fall when you hold her and say in a choked voice that it is "OK" if she can't accept that gift from you.

Once she agrees to try, you need to make it easier for her by making your semen tastier. Eating the proper foods before oral sex is very important. If a man eats certain fruits—particularly pineapples, citrus, and melon—before getting a blow job, his ejaculate will taste sweeter, while fatty foods and spicy foods will make it bitter. Alkaline-based foods such as meat and fish can produce a bitter, fishy taste; and dairy products, which contain a high bacterial content, create an unpleasant taste. Acidic foods such as sweets and fruits should give bodily fluids a pleasant, sugary flavor. However, alcohol drinkers should take care not to drink chemically processed liquors, as those can cause semen to have a very acidic taste. A vegetarian meal with plenty of acidic fruit and naturally fermented wines and spirits provides the best-tasting semen—but stay away from asparagus, broccoli, or beets, which can impart a bad taste. Vitamins, coffee, cigarettes, and garlic, as well as some "recreational" drugs such as cocaine, can also adversely affect the taste of the seminal fluid. Abstaining from these alkaline, dairy, and other "bad" foods and drinking plenty of water at least 24 hours before engaging in oral sex will go a long way toward making her more eager to swallow.

Finally, you should encourage her to swallow quickly and rapidly when she feels your cum in her throat. Not only will that mean there is less of a taste in her mouth but it also makes your orgasm that much more exciting from the suction of rapid swallowing. So quick gulps will increase both your pleasure and hers. Bon appétit!

TIP #32: To get her to swallow, convince her that your semen is the carrier of your life energy. On the day of the big event, make sure to drink plenty of water and eat lots of fruit to make sure your ejaculate taste better. Finally, encourage her to gulp it down fast—this way she'll hardly taste it! ✦

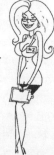

GETTING IN THE BACK DOOR,
OR "ANAL" FOR BEGINNERS

Many women cringe at the thought of anal sex. It's not usually because of any moral or religious objections; it is because anal sex can be painful even if performed properly. However, many women can learn to love anal sex if introduced to anal stimulation in a gentle and gradual manner. Pet of the Year Heather Vandeven said that she ended up trying anal sex because the guy she was with "was enthusiastic yet patient about it." Pet of the Year Runner-up Courtney Taylor echoes Heather's sentiments about anal sex. She says she tried it because her man "asked nicely, and I trusted him, and it was a long-term relationship." Pet of the Month Krista Ayne also tried anal because "he told me it would not hurt because he knew how to do it, but it still hurt . . . a lot." Julie Strain only had anal sex with her husband. She jokes she'd have it again "only if we stayed at the Plaza in New York. The treat of being treated really matters." So, patience and trust seem to be paramount when requesting anal sex from your hottie—and don't expect it unless you've been with her for a while.

To develop her curiosity about anal explorations, get Tony Bentley's ode to anal sex called *Surrender* or Alicia Erian's *The Gradual Approach* or rent the movie *Last Tango in Paris* and watch the famous "butter" scene from this controversial Bertolucci film that popularized anal sex. If she is willing to watch porn with you, you will have plenty of examples of women going ape over anal. Select the ones where the female stars "squirt" while being anally penetrated. That will prove positively to your own partner that anal can be exciting.

Use a little physical persuasion as well. While performing oral sex on her, finger or lick her perenium, the area between the vagina and the anus, and work your way down to the anus itself. Circle the outer rim of the anus with your finger or tongue. If she enjoys this stimulation, try manually caressing her anus during woman-on-top intercourse. Using Pavlovian conditioning, combining light anal stimulation with sexual activities that she finds pleasurable will create in her a mental association between anal stimulation and orgasm, making further explorations easier. Once she begins to enjoy the anal touch, you can penetrate her anus with a well-lubricated finger and slowly work your way toward substituting a cock for that finger. There are three steps in this process:

Step 1: Proper Lubrication

Before penetrating her anus, make sure you have the proper lubrication. Unlike the vagina, there is little or no natural lubrication in the anus; therefore, you must use commercial lubricants. Oil-based lubricants are the best for anal sex because they last longer, but the drawback for oil-based lubricants is that they will damage a latex-based condom. So if you plan to use a latex-based condom, use water-based lubricants and frequently reapply them.

Step 2: Fingering

Start with any finger other than the thumb or pinky because you want to have complete control over digital penetration. Circle the outer rim of the anus, making swirling motions. Next take one finger and push on the anus, as though you were ringing a doorbell. Push lightly, then harder, then hold down for a second or two before releasing. Insert your finger into the anus and wiggle it around, using a tapping motion, then move in and out with a thrusting motion, similar to penetration during sex. Try inserting one finger in her anus and one in her vagina and stimulate the shared walls between the vagina and the rectum. Just be careful not to switch the finger from the anus to the vagina or vice versa— you might even want to use different hands for anal and vaginal stimulation.

Step 3: Penetration

Once the anal sphincter is sufficiently relaxed through oral and digital stimulation and sufficiently lubricated, she should be ready for object and penile penetration. Some toys such as anal probes are specifically designed for loosening the sphincter and preparing for penile penetration. Encourage her to relax and breath outward during insertion. Do not stimulate other erogenous zones while attempting anal intercourse because it can cause inopportune sphincter contractions. Do not begin to pump right away, instead ease each little bit in and slowly withdraw until she can handle thrusting action. Once this is accomplished, she can intensify her pleasure sensations by contracting her anal muscles voluntarily in sync with involuntary contractions.

There is a common misconception that anal intercourse is easiest to accomplish in the doggie style position. Actually, the best position for anal penetration is missionary position with legs up because it allows her to relax the muscles necessary for pleasurable anal sex. Have her lie on her back, knees in the air. You should kneel or lie facing her, whichever is more comfortable for both of you. Another good beginner position is side anal, where she lies on her side and you approach her from the rear.

When you pull out, do it gently and gradually, as the sudden exit can make the sphincter muscles tense up and spasm more than usual.

TIP #33: To get her to try anal sex, you need to be extra patient and sensitive. Prepare her by gentle anal massage, then add a ton of lubricant and attempt anal fingering. Only after her anal sphincter muscle is fully relaxed should you attempt penetration very, very slowly. ✦

Three Makes a Party . . . Sometimes

As I mentioned in the chapter on fantasies, many women fantasize about having sex with multiple partners. I have to confess to having many such fantasies myself; and a lot of my model friends have admitted to similar "secret" desires. However, I have to warn you that fulfilling these fantasies is fraught with danger! Her fantasies, remember, are going to involve her having sex simultaneously with you and another guy; and you should be sure you are comfortable with that before even thinking of making that fantasy real. If there is even a tiny bit of potential jealousy or fear of competition or worry about losing her when you imagine her being with another guy, you shouldn't go there.

Your fantasies of having sex with your dream girl and another woman might be easier to pull off, especially if you find that your girl is bisexual or at least bi-curious and willing to try sex with another woman. However, even if she is willing, you have to proceed cautiously. If she develops jealousy at seeing your lust for another woman, it could be curtains for any future relationship.

Talking Her into It

Many guys believe that it is harder to talk a hot woman into a threesome than an average-looking one. In fact, most of the hot models I have worked with and interviewed had bisexual tendencies, and many have experimented with other women. Many women in the modeling and glamour world are used to changing in front of other women and seeing each other naked, so making out with other hot women is only logical. What you need to figure out is not how to talk her into being with another woman but how to convince her that you should be included!

According to my surveys, alcohol has a lot to do with centerfolds' decisions to try out a threesome, so having a relaxed, festive atmosphere and some booze as a disinhibitor seems to be a must. This is how Pet of the Month Krista Ayne describes her first threesome: "I was at a club with one of my friends and a guy I was dating. We were dancing, drinking, and having a really good time. After that we went back to his apartment to continue the party. I told them I wanted to play a drinking game where after every shot someone has to take off an item of clothing. Soon we were all half naked and I started kissing her. After that I told them we should go to his bed—you know what happened next." Of course, occasionally a hottie will have a threesome because she wants to do something nice for you. This is what Jamie Lynn did; "a friend was moving out of town and my girlfriend and I wanted to give him a going-away gift . . . in reality, we both wanted a piece of him, so why not do it together?"

Step 1: If You Don't Know If She Is into Chicks
(If You Do, Go to Step 2)

Start by initiating a general discussion of bisexuality in women. Mention that you read this study that said that most women get turned on by thoughts of being with other women. Watch *The L Word* with her or take her to see the movie *Kinsey*. Ask her if she agrees with the idea that women know best how to make love to another woman. If she does not volunteer having any lesbian experiences, ask her about any sexual fantasies she might have had about making love to another woman. If she is into watching or reading porn with you, pick a video or book with a hot girl-on-girl scene and get excited and amorous when that scene is on—you know you can do that! Tell her that you are imagining her in that scene. Or, if she is comfortable with your reading *Penthouse*, show her some recent issues and ask for her opinion on the sexiness of the Pets or other nude models pictured. Otherwise, wait until you see a hot chick when you are out together—pick one that meets HER description of the kind of woman that turns her on—and ask her whether the girl is sexy.

If she is even more adventurous, put a sexual "wish basket" next to your bed filled with your and her wishes. Take turns drawing from that basket and talking about—or acting out—each other's fantasies. Put "watching two women together" into the mix; and when it is drawn, tell her that that means you would like to see her with another woman. Or, tell her you want to go down on her while she imagines her favorite female icon doing it to her (for me, it would be Angelina Jolie); if she agrees, give her the best head of her life.

In other words, get her to thinking about how hot other women are; and then slide in the thought that she might like to make love to another woman and that you would love to see it. Make sure you always convey an assurance that you have no problem with female bisexuality and that you would never be jealous of her sleeping with another woman. On the other hand, if you find that she expresses religious or moral objections to lesbian sex, you might have to discard the whole idea—or find a new girl.

Step 2: If You Know She Is into Chicks

When you have gotten her to admit that she would like to try sex with another woman, you are ready for the next step. Remember, she has to feel safe and confident in your feelings for her, and she must believe that your relationship is on solid ground. Otherwise she is likely to feel too insecure to bring another woman into the mix. If she likes the idea of being with another woman but expresses discomfort with being watched, get her accustomed to the whole voyeuristic experience by setting up a mirror in your bedroom or videotaping you together. Tell her you'll destroy the tape afterwards—and really do that. Convince her that you would really like to watch her in bed with another woman because it would help you learn how to please her better. She will undoubtedly ask what you would do if you watched. Reply that you would either beat off or join in if she approved. Here is where you emphasize that you would only participate if she were comfortable with it, since your primary goal is to enhance HER pleasure and to enjoy a hot experience with HER. If she buys this line, you are ready to "negotiate" terms for a threesome. Actually, the terms are non-negotiable: she gets to pick out the other woman and to tell you in advance how far you can go in participating (i.e., only watching, only making out with the other woman, or only oral sex, or full intercourse but only after your girl has had you first, etc.). If she only allows watching, go for it, because you know she will get turned on by watching you masturbate and will likely invite you to join in anyway. Remember—her rules are subject to change at any time! At this point, it is only a matter of time before you will find yourself in a "chick sandwich!"

Warning: as I have said before, triangles are tricky. Don't expect to be the center of attention—instead, try to make your girl the "star" of the show. However, your girlfriend might discover that she likes the new dish so much that she might just put you out in the cold. And don't pay too much attention to the new girl—or you will lose the old one.

TIP #34: To get her to try ménage à trois, first find out if she is into other women by exploring her fantasies. If she is, convince her that you would really like to watch her in bed with another woman because it would help you learn how to please her better. Then let her set all the rules and choose a woman she would be comfortable with. Expect her to change the rules at any time! And make sure not to pay too much attention to the other woman! ✦

CHANGE YOUR SEXUAL SCRIPTS

Many hot women are sensation-seekers, which means they will look for greener pastures the minute your well of sexual tricks dries up. If you want to keep her feeling that butterflies-in-the-stomach feeling, throw caution to the wind and seek some sensual adventure. Comfort and familiarity are lust-killers, so if you want to keep her heart aflutter, and your penis a-pumping, you have to get that adrenaline going by injecting some new sensations into your sexual script:

1. Alfresco-sex. Don't just do her in your stuffy bedroom, get outdoors and get some back-to-nature nookie. The recirculated air in your home can cause drowsiness and fatigue, so air out your lungs and your genitals. It will literally and figuratively electrify your sex life—the oxygen molecule is negatively charged, and pumping your lungs full of O_2 will pump up your willy too. Also, soaking up some sun will boost your testosterone level and hers too. So make sure to bring an extra large blanket to your picnic, or a tent for that hike in the woods.

2. Aqua-sex. The feel of water against your body adds to the sensuality of liquid loving, and the way she looks dripping wet is an instantaneous turn-on too. Water also adds buoyancy to your body, allowing you to experiment with new positions. For these reasons, wet sex is often wild sex, so take your honey on a cruise—even if it's only in a pool or your bathtub. Nothing beats the allure of a romantic screw on the beach washed by the ocean waves, but if you cannot afford a tropical getaway, remind her that swimming pools are free of dangerous undercurrents, and hot tubs get her quickly hot and bothered with the aid of those water massagers. But remember, salty water is actually not the friendliest vaginal environment, and even fresh water can wash away the lubrication in the vagina, causing excess friction, so make sure to have some lube on hand. For the best in slippery sex, make sure she is as wet on the inside as she is on the outside!

3. Claustro-sex. Having sex in a confined place can offer an unexpected degree of physical intimacy. Remember the high school thrill of making out in your old compact car, her knees all the way up to her chin, and her feet on the steering wheel? Try making out in a telephone booth—before they go extinct due to cellular technology. If you are traveling to Great Britain, these dinosaurs are still alluringly bright red; and there is nothing like humping in a "limey red light district." For those of you who prefer a little more breathing room, try elevator sex—press the stop button and see if you can cum before security comes. Or see if you can get enough maneuverability in a sleeping bag—or go goth and do it in a coffin!

4. Transit-sex. We spend half our life commuting, so why not have some sex on the move? Have her practice her hand-job skills while the two of you are stuck in traffic in a car, or get it on in an empty subway car late at night. Or ride in the backseat of a bus and let the engine vibrations get her going. Then pretend to drop your wallet and park your head under her skirt. Then it's her turn to see if she can get you off before it's time to get off.

5. Alti-sex. Otherwise known as mile-high sex or sex at high altitude, it's most commonly practiced in the bathrooms of airplanes (in which case it's alti-claustro-sex!). Fortunately for those who fear that the flight attendant will be banging on the door while you are banging your girlfriend, there are other alternatives to get that head-spinning alti-sex feeling. For example, she'll love the giddy sensation of peering over a balcony while you are ramming her from behind. A little "edge-play" on the roof will get her heart (and your member) pumping and your heads spinning, so make sure you both have a firm grip on the railings. Then, for those with a little more guts—and cash—you can rent a hot air balloon for a more leisurely lay in the sky.

6. Exhibito-sex. Begin by having sex in front of mirrors, then masturbating her with your foot under the table at a restaurant, then get more brazen and try it any place where you may be seen. Movie theaters are perfect places to practice a little exhibitionism without sacrificing comfort. Pick an NC-17 feature, preferably a subtitled French film, and get busy in the plush back row. She might get so inspired that she would want to star in your own homemade productions (in which case it's exhibito-porno-sex).

7. Cell-sex. Women are not the only aural creatures—men are surprisingly responsive to dirty talk! And these days phone sex is also text-messaging sex. Here are some lines to get you started: KOTL (Kiss on the lips), KOTL> (Kiss on the love lips), I WaNU2Sckit (I want you to suck it). And don't forget UrTxtMMH (Your text makes me hard).

8. Role-play-sex. What girl hasn't fantasized about getting a gynecological exam from a handsome and perverse doctor? Role-play sex allows you to safely play out your dirtiest fantasies under the guise of make-believe. So go ahead, put on that robber mask and pretend to rape her—just make sure she knows you are playing a game!

9. BDSM-sex. You don't have to be a sadist to get into some spanking, pussy-smacking action, and trust me, virtually every girl loves to be restrained and ordered around (in bed, of course!). One of my fondest sexual memories is that of me naked, blindfolded, and strung out between two birch trees, with my boyfriend indulging in some serious ass-whipping foreplay with freshly stripped birch twigs. So get some restraints—whether they are your old ties, or toy handcuffs—and show her who is the boss.

10. Astro-sex. The intergalactic excursions will soon be open for business, so if you can afford it, why not practice your sex moves in microgravity? If you are wealthy, but not rich enough for cosmo-sex, there is a gravity-free bed created by a Dutch designer that hovers in midair with the aid of powerful magnets. The only drawback is the price—about 1.2 million euros. For the rest of us, there are always imitations, such as a good ole' sex swing.

Twenty-four

Afterglow: Fighting the Urge to Turn Over and Snore

Come, cuddle your head on my shoulder, dear
Your head like the golden-rod,
And we will go sailing away from here
To the beautiful land of Nod.

—ELLA WHEELER WILCOX

If you are like most men, you have a tendency to want to roll over and go to sleep after sex. If you have that tendency, you have probably heard some carping from your partner—and if you haven't yet, you will. Next to bad oral skills and an inability to last long enough, the seeming inability of men to provide some postcoital loving is one of the top complaints that almost all women have.[65] If you want to be regarded as the best lover your honey has ever had, you simply must avoid spoiling the effect of all your skills by neglecting her needs in this critical "afterglow" period.

In your defense, there is a physiological reason that many men feel sleepy after orgasm, and this is because the postclimactic blood rush depletes the muscles of energy-producing glycogen, leaving them feeling physically drained. Glycogen loss also triggers the release of adenosine, which acts as a messenger to the cells, triggering sleep. Because men have more muscle mass than women, men are more likely to feel sleepy just when their partners are yearning for some après-sex cuddling.

On the other hand, a woman's body demands cuddling, thanks to her unique chemistry. In both men and women, an orgasm triggers the release of oxytocin, a hormone that promotes closeness, intimacy, and even love by making the person feel all "warm and fuzzy" in the presence of the partner who has triggered the oxytocin flood. These feelings of "glowing" with warmth and happiness are what give the postclimax period the name "afterglow." Oxytocin is one of the most powerful hormones in the human body; it may well be the chemical foundation of human beings' being able to live together in harmony and to build group, clan, and family relationships. However, the female body produces *50 percent more oxytocin* after an orgasm than does a male body, so while you might experience a brief wash of such feelings lasting a minute or so, she is experiencing these feelings twice as strongly as you do and for much longer.

Moreover, female sexuality is closely tied to oxytocin release, as it is mediated by estrogen, the primary female sexual hormone. (Men have some estrogen in their bodies too but their sex drive is mostly controlled by testosterone.) For example, women get the same oxytocin "rush" from breast-feeding as they do from orgasm, because both nursing and sex are, for her, estrogen-regulated events. Indeed, evolution has "locked in" a direct connection between sex and mate attachment in a woman's mind, due to her need to bind her partner to her to protect her and her children. Thus, for a woman, the emotional feelings induced by oxytocin are just as important, if not more important, than the number and intensity of the orgasms she experiences.

Therefore, to make your sexual encounters really pleasurable for your partner, you simply have to shake off that sleepiness long enough to give her a good after-sex cuddling. It's not hard to do,

after all. You're both naked, and the body that attracted you to her
in the first place is right there to be caressed and stroked. That
face that stunned you with its beauty and made you choose her to
approach that first day is right next to yours, begging to be kissed.
There is no chemical or psychological pressure on you at this
point, as your body has just had a great orgasm. It's time to let your
hands leisurely explore those voluptuous curves, and to let your
lips gently pay homage to her eyes, her smile, and even her cute
little nose. A little "pillow talk" is also in order here: some sweet
romantic thoughts, if that is what you are feeling for her, or at least
some genuine words of appreciation for her sharing these pleasurable moments with you. Eventually, she will start to feel sleepy, too,
as the languor of her limbs spreads throughout her body; then you
can let her go. But until then, keep all your attention on her and
make sure she remembers those moments as particularly precious
memories of your lovemaking.

If you have trouble fighting off sleep, there are several ways you
can deal with it. One of the best is to get up, go to the bathroom,
and get her a warm, wet washcloth and a drying towel to wipe the
sweat and any love juices from her body, especially her genitals.
Even if you've used a condom, there is going to be unwanted moisture to mop up; and if you've gone "bareback," there is definitely a
need to negate the "wet spot" before it occurs. Since a woman who
has just climaxed is often jelly-legged, weak, and even a little disoriented for a while afterwards, this is a duty that falls to you. While
you are at it, you can—after washing your own genitals—splash a
little water in your face, or do a few quick exercises, or whatever
it takes to shake off your drowsiness. Then, after you have gently
washed and dried her, you can pull up the covers and take her in
your arms for the cuddling she craves.

Other sleep-avoidance techniques could include popping a stimulating CD in your stereo, getting the both of you a drink (you will
be a little dehydrated after vigorous sex), and opening a window to
get some cool, fresh air on your face. Whatever it takes, and what-

ever works, you should do, because making the postcoital period good for her is just as important as delivering on your orgasm promise.

"Pillow talk time" is also a good time to be paying attention to her for an additional reason. After a stunning climax and a sweet cuddle, she will likely be more open and honest in her thoughts than she would be at any other time. So it's a good time to find out about her sexual fantasies, her feelings about sex, love, and men (in general—never force her to compare), and her dreams and aspirations. Oxytocin also inspires trust, so not only will she be more open but she will also more likely to believe what you tell her. This is the time when you can reinforce all the things about yourself that you want her to believe, as well as gain insight into her inner thoughts and feelings, so that you can decide where you want your relationship to go. For many couples, this postcoital "pillow talk time" is the most meaningful time in their relationship. You should make it yours too!

Top 10 Things to Do During Afterglow

1. Get her a washcloth

2. Hold her

3. Get her a drink

4. Snack on something

5. Take a shower together

6. Daydream

7. Listen to music

8. Watch a video

9. Give back or foot massages

10. Play an adult board game

When You Wake Up beside Her

The glances over cocktails,
That seem to be so sweet,
Don't seem quite so amorous,
Over Shredded Wheat.   —FRANK MUIR

Some men seem to be great lovers at night but monsters in the morning. I have dumped quite a few guys in my life because they acted like selfish, insensitive jerks on the morning after our first sexual encounter. If you want this hottie that you have wooed and wowed into your bed to be more than a one-night stand, you can't just throw away your success when the morning sunlight streams in. Instead, you want to set the stage for your next night together, whether it be right away or a week later.

In some sense, acting dumbly in the a.m. is understandable. I am not a "morning person," and a lot of my model friends also are not at their best at the crack of dawn—or even the crack of noon! If your honey is like me, she will awaken with sleepy, droopy eyes, frizzy or messed-up hair, and a few wrinkles that you didn't notice before, as they were covered by makeup. If you didn't shower or take a bath (hopefully together) after your sex bout or bouts the night before, she might have lingering odors of sweat or even love fluids clinging to her skin. So she won't necessarily look like the perfect goddess you might have thought she was when she was all made up and looking her best for you. But then, neither will you!

However, because she knows that she doesn't look her best in the morning, she will be extrasensitive about her looks and what you think of her. This is not a time for "fat" jokes or snide remarks about her mussy hair. Every negative thing you say in these moments will be multiplied by her own angst about letting you see, likely for the first time, her un-made-up face and unprepared body in broad daylight. Making her uncomfortable about letting you see the "real thing" will only lead to a future unwillingness to undergo the experience again. Instead, this is another key time when you need to give her MAJOR reassurances as to her beauty and desirability.

Every guy who has made me want to stay with him, or even move in with him, has been a guy who has paid me compliments about my frizzy morning hair ("It's so sexy to see that 'bedroom hair,' which reminds me of what a passionate time we had last night"), or my naked, unadorned face ("You know, you look even more beautiful without makeup"). Not that I believed these statements, because I don't think I look that great in the morning, but I loved the guy for trying to make me feel good. And when after I bitched about my disheveled looks, he pulled me into his arms and gave me a soft, sweet "morning kiss"—even though I hadn't brushed my teeth as yet—I knew that I had made the right choice to sleep with him.

That is what you want your girl to feel too. You don't have to lay it on thick; just be as appreciative of her charms in the daylight as you were the night before. But be sure she knows how much you like the way she looks and how sexy she is. Prove it with a touch, a kiss, and some genuine smiles. If she encourages you, and you aren't in a rush, turn those morning kisses into a prelude to another round of lovemaking. In my experience, sex in the morning, when you feel refreshed and full of energy, and can see the looks in each other's eyes and admire each other's bodies by daylight, is even better than the usual kind of bedtime sex. However, even if you don't have the time or the energy for another round, make her believe you want to. That way, she'll have another reason to come back to your bed another night. And if, in fact, she gives you the line "Yeah, it's too bad you and I have to go to work now; but maybe another time . . ." make a date for that "other time" right then and there. (Remember, though, that if you are still in the early phases of your relationship, you don't want to appear too eager or available, so make it for a few days off.)

Another way in which guys turn off their bedmates when the

sun is up is by acting too "cocky" and full of themselves after their "conquest" of the night before. One of the things women fear the most, even the most beautiful of women, is that if they go to bed with a man, he will come to think of them as "a piece of ass," or just another sexual object. Any kind of behavior that suggests that this is how you regard her, whether it be bragging about how good you were in bed, or how many orgasms you gave her, or any comparisons of her to other women, is going to spoil the party for your chosen hottie. A cool, suave Prince Charming–type never brags, exults, or makes any kind of reference to his performance in bed— especially to the woman who has experienced that performance. He is confident that his skills speak for themselves. If she gives him a compliment about his lovemaking, he smiles and gives her a throw-away line like "Thanks, but sex is even better when a couple gets to know each other well, so I'm sure you'll think even better of me in the future." Always leave her wanting more!

If she makes the silly mistake of asking you for your opinion of *her* skills in bed, you must never give her a negative opinion—even if she was a dud who just lay there and let you do everything. If she was so bad you don't want her back, you will not invite her back; but you want her feeling good about you anyway. Hey, she might be your entrée to her hottie girlfriend who is more of a tigress in bed! So find a way to compliment her, no matter what you really think. As one of my male friends put it, "If I can't think of anything else nice to say, I'll tell her that I loved the way she cried out and shook when she came—'real passion,' I'd describe it—so that she would be eager to get to that moment again."

Finally, if you want her to continue seeing you and giving her all to you in bed, you should continue to treat her in the morning with the same respect, attitudes, and behavior as you did the night, or the date, before. If you are the breakfast-making kind, and have the time, by all means make her a good breakfast. But if Starbucks or a McMuffin is your idea of breakfast, you should tell her that and invite her along if she has the time, but do not alter your own morning routine overly much just to suit her. Yes, you have now had sex with her; however, being the self-confident alpha male, you fully expected that. No matter how many flip-flops your heart might be doing in a state of limerence, you will never let her know it. While you have now entered into a new phase of your relationship—as lovers—you haven't changed in any essential way, so continue the "capture her heart" or "get her to bed" techniques that have been successful thus far. The fact that you had sex with her, even drove her crazy in orgasmic paroxysms, and yet remain calm and collected and unruffled by the experience will make her want you more. So, when the time comes, take her home or to her car, thank her for a wonderful evening and night, and give her a nice kiss—and, if you still want her, promise to call her soon.

That promise to call her "soon" is the one way your program will change after you have bedded her. By sleeping with you, and giving you reason to believe she would do it again, she has shown you that she is definitely interested in you as a possible romantic partner—sex for a woman always involves this implied outcome—but that has left her vulnerable. If you are too aloof and "unavailable" now, she is going to jump to the conclusion that you have no romantic interest in her, and rather than get hurt, she will want to break it off right away. Whether you do or do not see her as a potential full-time girlfriend, if you want to keep seeing her, you must demonstrate your interest in her with the frequency that she will expect from a potential partner. Most of my girlfriends say that means calling at least several times a week—for me, it would be every other day at a minimum!—and taking her out, with or without sex, at least weekly.

To keep her from thinking you are only interested in sex, you should plan some dates where it won't be on the schedule: lunch dates, meetings where you help her get her car fixed, quick dinners at or near her office or yours when either of you have to work late, daytime shopping trips (when you don't have time to spend the night), etc. But to keep her as a sexual partner, you will also work in a fair number of more romantic dates, where you can expect to end the night in bed. In due course, you will want to plan some romantic weekend getaways, to a bed-and-breakfast in a quaint or secluded locale, to your parents' cabin at the shore or in the mountains (without them, of course), or any similar place you can afford. If you want to test your compatibility first, you can propose an entire weekend in your bed—and make it special with catered or pre-prepared meals, flowers by the bedside, champagne in the fridge, and a brand-new sexy negligee in her favorite color for her to wear. If you are still hot for each other after 48 hours of nonstop sex and intimate conversation, then you no longer need this book!

Tip from the Scoring Experts *Duke Ellington, the great bandleader and musician, charmed women with his soulful bedroom eyes and carefree attitude. Always flashily dressed (his nickname came from his elegant attire), the Duke affected a truly gallant pose, with hand kissing, flowers on his piano, and gifts upon parting with each of his paramours. He made his conquests each feel that they were special, with theatrical flourishes to add to their impression that a night with the Duke was the greatest moment in their lives.*

Afterword

She walks in beauty, like the night / Of cloudless climes and starry skies; / And all that's best of dark and bright / Meet in her aspect and her eyes.
—LORD BYRON

Man is the hunter, woman is his game:
The sleek and shining creatures of the chase,
We hunt them for the beauty of their skins.
—ALFRED LORD TENNYSON

You have dreamed of her, maybe worshipped her in your mind, and perhaps masturbated to her pictures or to the mental images you can't get out of your head. But you have always doubted that you had what it took to actually meet her, win her affections, and wake to find her cuddled by your side. But, after reading this book, I hope you have cast your doubts aside. The hottest women are not unattainable—far from it. Many of them have trouble getting dates from guys they would really like to go out with, because so many such guys are too afraid to ask, or if they do, they stumble and fall over their ignorance of how to handle a hot woman. Yet for every hot model that falls in love with, or marries, a movie or rock star or some rich dude, there are two who marry guys with ordinary jobs, decent but not spectacular looks, and no particular reputation with women. Indeed, one Playmate I know, whose every fan thinks her unapproachable, married a very average-looking UPS deliveryman!

But while you may be average in looks, in income, or in other respects, if you have read this book and assimilated its contents, you are *not* an average guy when it comes to handling hot women. You have in your hands the latest scientifically tested, verifiable psychological advice from a super-centerfold who has heard every line and been the object of every form of seduction that has ever found its way into print. The techniques in this book work with any hottie I've ever met. They would even work with me if I didn't know you were using the "Dr. Z method" on me—and even if I did know, I'd probably be impressed enough at your seductive skills that I would go out with you anyway!

So now it's up to you to use this advice to make your dreams come true. You can't make any more excuses. Dr. Z has told you in no uncertain terms that you have what it takes to hit on the hottie of your choice, and how to score, and she has shown you how to do it. Prove me right!

VICTORIA ZDROK, PH.D.
Penthouse Pet of the Year;
Playboy Playmate

Dr. Z's Scoring Program

Construct your love map by analyzing the type of women you like.

Keep in mind the fact that hot women are insecure, neurotic, high-maintenance, entitled, picky, and yearn to be more than mere sex objects.

Decide what popular prototype you want to emulate by analyzing your own image.

Serendipity Approach

Seek out natural habitats of your prototypical hottie.

Be on the lookout for chance encounters.

Propinquity Approach

Create a sense of familiarity by frequenting that habitat or infiltrating it.

Get Her Attention

Project dominance.

Imitate her movements.

Ditch your nerdy buddy.

Dress stylishly and in accordance with prototype. Wear blue when in doubt.

Improve your voice by lowering pitch and enunciating.

Work on your grooming, attend to dental hygiene and physical exercise. Use pheromones to increase your appeal.

Develop Self-Confidence

• List your positive traits

• Develop internal locus of control

• Learn unconditional self-acceptance

• Visualize yourself as confident

• Replace negative thoughts with positive ones

• Stop "musturbation" and "shoulding"

• Emphasize effort, not outcome

• See uncertainty as a challenge

Reaching Rejection Immunity State (RIS)

• Stop "catastrophizing" and "awfullizing"

• Challenge your anxiety with logic

• Find humor in the situation

• Demystify beauty

• Practice, practice, practice!

Cultivate and Display other Values
that Appeal to Women

- Humor/wit

- Magnanimity/kindness

- Equanimity/stability

- Ambition/industriousness

- Chivalry/courtesy

- Independence/autonomy

- Intelligence/erudition

- Spontaneity/risk taking

Notes

1. Robert Greene, *The Art of Seduction*. New York: Penguin Books, 2003.

2. Asch, S. (1946). "Forming Impressions of Personality." *Journal of Abnormal and Social Psychology*, 41, 258–290.

3. Why does this happen? Because of the so-called primacy effect, which makes us pay more attention to the information we receive first. Once we have some initial information at our disposal, we just don't bother to pay a lot of attention to additional input. We tend to be what psychologists call "cognitive misers"—we do the least amount of cognitive work we can in thinking about others.

4. Dawkins, R. *The Selfish Gene*. Oxford: Oxford University Press, 1976.

5. Buss, D. M., and Dedden, L. A. (1990). "Derogation of Competitors." *Journal of Social and Personal Relationships*, 7, 395–422.

6. Ford, C.S., and Beach, F. A. *Patterns of Sexual Behavior*. New York: Harper & Row, 1951.

7. Campbell, Kim. "Today's Courtship: White Teeth, Root Beer and E-mail?" February, 14, 2002. *The Christian Science Monitor*.

8. Moore, C. (Mar, 20, 2002). "Increased Sex Appeal, by a Nose Pheromones Work, Study Says." *The Atlanta Journal*.

9. Shorey, H. H. *Animal Communication by Pheromones*. New York: Academic Press, 1976.

10. Ford, C. S., and Beach, F. A. *Patterns of Sexual Behavior*. New York: Harper & Row, 1951.

11. One2One living, one2onemag.com, Vol. 02, No. 03, p. 17.

12. Buss, D. M. *The Evolution of Desire, Strategies of Human Mating.* rev. ed. New York: Basic Books/Perseus Book Group, 2003.

13. Csikszentmihalyi, Mihaly. *The Psychology of Optimal Experience.* New York: Harper Perennial, 1991.

14. Townsend, John M., and Levy, Gary D. (1990). "Effects of Potential Partner's Physical Attractiveness and Socioeconomic Status on Sexuality and Partner Selection." *Archives of Sexual Behavior,* 19 (2), 149–164.

15. Hill, E. M., Nocks, E. S., and Gardner, L. (1987). "Physical Attractiveness: Manipulation by Physique and Status Displays." *Ethology and Sociobiology,* 8, 143–154.

16. Greene, *The Art of Seduction,* p. 104.

17. Zajonc, R. B., Murphy, S. T., and Inglehart, M. (1989). "Feeling and Facial Efference: Implication of the Vascular Theory of Emotion." *Psychological Review,* 96, 395–416.

18. Isen, A. M., Daubman, K. A., and Nowicki, G. P. (1987). "Positive Affect Facilitates Creative Problem Solving." *Journal of Personality and Social Psychology,* 52, 1122–1131.

19. Ellis, A. (2003). "Early Theories and Practices of Rational Emotive Behavior Theory and How They Have Been Augmented and Revised During the Last Three Decades." *Journal of Rational-Emotive & Cognitive-Behavior Therapy,* 21 (3/4).

20. Maslow, A. *Motivation and Personality.* 3rd ed. New York: HarperCollins, 1987.

21. Cloyd, J. W. (1976). "The Market-place Bar: The Interrelation between Sex, Situation, and Strategies in the Pairing Ritual of Homo Ludens." *Urban Life,* 5, 293–312. Nesse, R. M. (1990).

22. Botwin, M. D., Muss, D. M., and Shakelford, T. K. (1997). "Personality and Mate Preferences: Five Factors in Mate Selection and Marital Satisfaction." *Journal of Personality,* 65 (1), 107–36.

23. Feingold, A. (1992). "Gender Differences in Mate Selection Preferences: A Test of the Parental Investment Model." *Psychological Bulletin,* 112 (1), 125–39.

24. Hamida, B. S., Mineka, S., and Bailey, J. M. (1998). "Sex Differences

in Perceived Controllability of Mate Value: An Evolutionary Perspective." *Journal of Personality and Social Psychology,* 75 (4), 953–66.

25. Why are humor and wit so important in the mate selection process? One quick answer is that laughter causes us to release endorphins, the happy hormones, thus making us feel good; and that good feeling extends to the bringer of laughter. Another answer is that smiling and laughter signify warmth, friendliness, and a pleasant disposition—all qualities that make a person likeable. Also, being able to see the lighter side of things implies an ability to enjoy life and to have fun; and the hottest women all like to have fun—indeed, some of them look at having fun as a main goal in life! Certainly, being quick-witted and funny is the opposite of being boring and dull, and no woman likes a dullard by her side. Finally, an ability to make a refined humorous remark also requires intelligence, self-confidence, and spontaneity, all of which are traits that women appreciate in men.

26. Greene, *The Art of Seduction,* pp. 133–134.

27. Ford, C. S., and Beach, F. A. *Patterns of Sexual Behavior.* New York: Harper & Row, 1951.

28. Why is kindness so important to women? Kindness signals a guy's ability and willingness to commit energy and resources to them and to have empathy with potential children that the relationship might bear. Even if a woman is not thinking of a long-term relationship or children when she meets you, her subconscious has those issues in tow. Female sexuality—what turns a woman on—is very closely related to her maternal drive; and in the back of her mind, every move she makes in the sexual or dating arena is judged by her ultimate maternal desires, the desires which have been honed by millions of years of evolution. Never forget this fact when you are trying to impress a woman: your suitability as a provider and father is always at issue, and anything you do should be directed at enhancing those potentials in her mind.

29. Buss, *The Evolution of Desire.* (When men were shown slides of a woman in the same three conditions, their attraction toward the woman was the same regardless of the condition.)

30. The reason intelligence is valued so highly by women is that it is correlated with higher income, better parenting skills, per-

spective-taking, communication, judgment, social adeptness, and problem-solving ability. Of the different types of intelligence, the one most valued by women is emotional intelligence, which consists of interpersonal (understanding your own needs and desires) and intrapersonal (sensitivity to needs and desires of others) intelligence.

31. Botwin, M. D., Muss, D. M., and Shakelford, T. K. (1997). "Personality and Mate Preferences: Five Factors in Mate Selection and Marital Satisfaction." *Journal of Personality*, 65 (1), 107–36.

32. Greene, *The Art of Seduction*, p. 191.

33. Zajonc, R. B. (1968). "Attitudinal Effects of Mere Exposure." *Journal of Personality and Social Psychology*, Monographs Supplement, 9–27.

34. Greene, *The Art of Seduction*, p. 178.

35. Knapp, M. L. *Nonverbal Communication in Human Interaction*. New York: Holt, Rinehart, & Winston, 1978.

36. Montepare, J. M., and Zebrowitz-McArthur, L. (1988). "Impressions of People Created by Age-Related Qualities of Their Gaits." *Journal of Personality and Social Psychology*, 54, 547–556.

37. Geiselman, R. E., Haight, N.A., and Kimata, L.G. (1984). "Context Effects on the Perceived Physical Attractiveness of Faces." *Journal of Experimental Social Psychology*, 2, 409–424.

38. Wedell, D. H., Parducci, A., and Geiselman, R. E. (1987). "A Formal Analysis of Ratings of Physical Attractiveness: Successive Contrast and Simultaneous Assimilation." *Journal of Experimental Social Psychology*, 23, 230–249.

39. Kleinke, C. L. (1986). "Gaze and Eye Contact: A Research Review." *Psychological Review*, 100, 78–100.

40. Strom, J. C., and Buck, R. W. (1979). "Staring and Participants' Sex: Physiological and Subjective Reactions." *Personality and Social Psychology Bulletin*, 5, 114–117.

41. Ellsworth, P. C., and Carlsmith, J. M. (1973). "Eye Contact and Gaze Aversion in Aggressive Encounter." *Journal of Personality and Social Psychology*, 33, 117–122.

42. Kleinke, C. L., Meeker, F. B., and Staneski, R. A. (1986). "Preference

for Opening Lines: Comparing Ratings by Men and Women." *Sex Roles,* 15, 585–600.

43. Feingold, A. (1989). "Gender Differences in Effects of Attractiveness and Similarity on Opposite-Sex Interaction: Integration of Self-Report and Experimental Findings." Unpublished manuscript, Yale University, New Haven, CT.

44. McAllister, H. A., and Bergman, N. J. (1983). "Self-Disclosure and Liking: An Integration Theory Approach." *Journal of Personality,* 51, 202–212.

45. Cloyd, J.W. (1976). "The Market-place Bar: The Interrelation between Sex, Situation, and Strategies in the Pairing Ritual of Homo Ludens." *Urban Life,* 5, 293–312, p. 300.

46. Fisher, H. *Why We Love: The Nature and Chemistry of Romantic Love.* New York: Henry Holt and Co., 2004.

47. In one study subjects were shown pictures of men and women in various settings. The same individuals were judged as more attractive when they were seated in a prettier room, better decorated with paintings and draperies. This demonstrates that we tend to transfer our feelings about our surroundings to the person we are with. Maslow, A. H., and Mintz, N. L. (1956). "Effects of Aesthetic Surroundings." *Journal of Psychology,* 41, 247–254.

48. Psychological research has shown that when subjects are well compensated for performing a task, they tend to rate the task as less enjoyable, attributing their desire to do the task to the compensation. When, on the other hand, the subjects are paid little or no compensation for doing the task, they are more likely to rate the task as enjoyable—why, otherwise, would they be doing it?

49. In one experiment, groups of male subjects were assigned to cross a cavern either using a steady, solid bridge or an unsteady, swaying one. The men were then shown a picture by a female research assistant and asked to come up with a story related to the picture. The men that crossed the shaky bridge wrote sexier stories and were much more likely to call the female experimenter at home to discuss the experience. Dutton, D. G., and Aron, A. P. (1974). "Some Evidence for Heightened Sexual Attraction under Conditions of High Anxiety." *Journal of Personality and Social Psychology,* 30, 510–517.

50. Ibid. In another study, men who were told that they would receive painful shocks as part of the research study rated the female confederate as more attractive than those who were told to expect only mild shocks.

51. A woman can effortlessly speak an average of 6,000 to 8,000 words a day. She uses an additional 2,000 to 3,000 vocal sounds to communicate, as well as 8,000 to 10,000 facial expressions, head movements, and other body language signals. This gives her a daily average of more than 20,000 communications. That explains why the British Medical Associates recently reported that women are four times more likely to suffer from jaw problems. Pease, Allan and Barbara. *Why Men Don't Listen & Women Can't Read Maps.* New York: Broadway Books, 2001, pp. 80–81.

52. It has just been discovered that women enjoy an oxytocin release (the cuddle and intimacy feeling hormone) from conversation alone— perhaps as a result of the way women bonded for companionship and protection when their menfolk were out on a hunt in prehistoric times. This release is triggered by estrogen in her body, so it isn't a benefit men normally enjoy (with the exception of lawyers, perhaps).

53. Byrne, D. *The Attraction Paradigm.* New York: Academic Press, 1971.

54. When a human experiences sexual attraction or lust, the brain releases adrenaline, which revs up the sympathetic nervous system responsible for faster breathing and heartbeat and slows down the parasympathetic nervous system responsible for digestion.

55. Greene, *The Art of Seduction,* p. 164.

56. When a reward is delayed in coming, the tardy delivery prolongs the activity of dopamine cells, speeding more of this natural stimulant into reward centers of the brain. Schultz, W. (2000). "Multiple Reward Signals in the Brain." Nature reviews. *Neuroscience,* 199–207.

57. This phenomenon is called the "cognitive consistency theory," as we all actively strive to be consistent in our attitudes, beliefs, and behaviors. Whenever inconsistency arises, we try to reconcile it with our convictions.

58. Greene, *The Art of Seduction,* p. 283.

59. Greene, *The Art of Seduction,* p. 434.

60. Lehrner, J., Eckersberger, C., Walla, P., Potsch, G., and Deecke, L. (2000). "Ambient Odor of Orange in a Dental Office Reduces Anxiety and Improves Mood in Female Patients." *Physiological Behavior*, 71(1–2): 83–6.

61. Women feel greater sexual desire and are much more likely to initiate sexual encounters during their ovulation.

62. When properly stimulated, a woman's breasts (and to some extent, male breasts as well) will likely undergo changes. Her nipples typically become erect and may become hard during sexual excitement. As excitement proceeds, the areolas begin to swell, continuing to the point where the earlier nipple erection may look less pronounced. The veins in the breast often become more visible as a result of the increased blood flowing into them, and there may also be a small increase in breast size.

63. Barbara Keesling. *Sexual Healing; The Complete Guide to Overcoming Common Sexual Problems*. Alameda, CA: Hunter House, 3rd Ed., 2006.

64. Sexologist Edward Eichel first described CAT in the early 1990s, but experienced lovers have used the method since the days of the Kama Sutra.

65. In a study of sex differences women reported a significantly greater preference for foreplay and afterplay than men. *Sex Differences in Sexual Needs and Desires*. Archives of Sexual Behavior, volume 13 (1984).

ABOUT THE AUTHOR

Not your ordinary dating expert, Dr. Victoria Zdrok is a unique and unprecedented combination of beauty, brains, brawn and . . . more beauty. The only woman to be both Playboy Playmate and Penthouse Pet of the Year, she holds a J.D. in law and a Ph.D. in clinical psychology. A self-described bookworm who turned to modeling to finance her education, Victoria managed to excel in both show business and academia, defying the stereotype of a blond bombshell and becoming a sex symbol and sexpert in one.

Born in Kiev, Ukraine, Victoria always dreamed of coming to America. Raised by anti-Communist parents, she diligently studied English with the hope of following that dream; at the age of 16, she became the first Soviet teenager allowed to come to the United States as a high school exchange student. Academic excellence helped Victoria receive her bachelors degree in psychology at the age of eighteen, and at nineteen she was accepted into a prestigious joint law and psychology graduate program hosted by Villanova Law School and Drexel University. She received her J.D. degree in law, became a member of the New York and New Jersey Bar Associations, and received her M.A., and then her Ph.D., in clinical psychology in 2003. Relentless in her intellectual pursuits, Victoria has also completed her postdoctorate certification in sex therapy under the direction of prominent sex therapist Dr. Sandra Leiblum at Robert Wood Johnson Medical School.

Concurrent with her academic career, Dr. Zdrok managed to have a flourishing career as a model. Discovered by a Playboy scout in her second year of law school, she became *Playboy*'s Miss October 1994. She also posed for *Penthouse*, and in June 2002, became Penthouse Pet of the Month and, in 2004, Penthouse Pet of the Year. In addition to her pinup work, Victoria has numerous credits as a model for bridal fashions, lingerie, and romance covers, as a featured guest on radio and TV shows, as an actress in commercials and movies, and as a spokesmodel for many products and services.

Besides her popularity as a smart sex symbol, Dr. Victoria Z has gained notoriety as a sexpert, dating coach, and relationship advisor through her magazine articles, television appearances, and radio interviews. She writes a monthly column for *Penthouse* magazine entitled "Ask Dr. Z" on love, sex, and dating, and a column for *Penthouse Forum*, which deals with sexuality and the law. She is a frequent contributor to a number of print and online publications, and the author of *Anatomy of Pleasure: The Head to Toe Guide to Better Sex.* Dr. Zdrok has her own Sirius Satellite Radio show on Howard 100, "The Sex Connection," and has been profiled on a number of entertainment journals and shows, as well as being a resident sexpert on Fox News. Dr. Z is currently developing her own sex education show, and her ultimate dream is to become the "Dr. Ruth of the Twenty-first century." You can find out more about Dr. Z on her site, www.SexySexpert.com. If you are interested in learning more about Dr. Z's dating advice, check out another of her websites, www.CourtshipTraining.com.